Neurological Clinical Examination

This book and video collection provide a practical guide to the clinical neurological examination, an essential tool in the diagnosis of neurological conditions encountered in the outpatient clinic and hospital ward.

- Each chapter covers a different condition and uses a step-by-step approach in selecting those aspects of the clinical examination which are most likely to lead to the correct diagnosis.

- Video clips accessible via both a companion website and by QR codes within the book provide easy access to view a wide range of neurological signs.

- The text is illustrated with clear diagrams.

- Tables are used to list the various causes of particular signs.

Primary care physicians, neurologists and trainees preparing for certifying examinations will find this book an invaluable learning companion and essential tool for the diagnosis of neurological disorders.

Neurological Clinical Examination

A Concise Guide

Fourth Edition

John Morris DM (OXON) FRACP FRCP
Emeritus Consultant, Westmead Hospital
Past Clinical Professor, University of Sydney
Past Chairman of the Education and Training Committee of the Australian and
New Zealand Association of Neurologists
Past Examiner for the Royal Australasian College of Physicians
Past Head of the Neurology Department, Westmead Hosptial
Past President of the Australian Association of Neurologists, Sydney, Australia

Joseph Jankovic MD
Professor of Neurology
Distinguished Chair in Movement Disorders
Director, Parkinson's Disease Center and Movement Disorders Clinic
Co-Director, Parkinson's Disease Research Laboratory
Past President of the Movement Disorders Society
Department of Neurology, Baylor College of Medicine, Houston, Texas, USA

Victor Fung MBBS (Hons) PhD FRACP
Conjoint Associate Professor, Sydney Medical School, University of Sydney
Director, Movement Disorders Unit, Department of Neurology, Westmead Hospital
Past Head, Department of Neurology, Westmead Hospital
Chair, Asia Pacific Affairs Committee, Australian and New Zealand Association of Neurologists
President-Elect, International Parkinson and Movement Disorder Society
Sydney, Australia

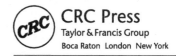

CRC Press
Taylor & Francis Group
Boca Raton London New York

CRC Press is an imprint of the
Taylor & Francis Group, an **informa** business

Fourth edition published 2023
by CRC Press
6000 Broken Sound Parkway NW, Suite 300, Boca Raton, FL 33487-2742

and by CRC Press
4 Park Square, Milton Park, Abingdon, Oxon, OX14 4RN

CRC Press is an imprint of Taylor & Francis Group, LLC

© 2023 Taylor & Francis Group, LLC

Library of Congress Cataloging-in-Publication Data
Names: Morris, John G. L., author. | Jankovic, Joseph, author. | Fung, Victor S. C., author.
Title: Neurological clinical examination : a concise guide / John GL Morris, Joseph Jankovic, Victor Fung.
Description: Fourth edition. | Boca Raton, FL : CRC Press, 2023. | Includes bibliographical references and index.
Identifiers: LCCN 2022017693 (print) | LCCN 2022017694 (ebook) | ISBN 9780367634353 (hardback) |
ISBN 9780367556129 (paperback) | ISBN 9781003119166 (ebook)
Subjects: MESH: Neurologic Examination--methods | Nervous System Diseases--diagnosis
Classification: LCC RC346 (print) | LCC RC346 (ebook) | NLM WL 141 | DDC 616.8/0475--dc23/eng/20220801
LC record available at https://lccn.loc.gov/2022017693
LC ebook record available at https://lccn.loc.gov/2022017694

ISBN: 978-0-367-63435-3 (hbk)
ISBN: 978-0-367-55612-9 (pbk)
ISBN: 978-1-003-11916-6 (ebk)

DOI: 10.1201/9781003119166

Typeset in Minion
by SPi Technologies India Pvt Ltd (Straive)

The cover image shows a vertical close-up view of David's hand from the famous statue of David by Italian sculptor Michelangelo.

Access the companion website: https://www.routledge.com/cw/morris

To study … disease without books is to sail an uncharted sea, while to study books without patients is not to go to sea at all.

William Osler
William B. Bean (ed.) (1950) *Sir William Osler Aphorisms*.
Henny Schuman, Inc., New York. p. 76.

Contents

List of videos ix

Foreword to the Third Edition xiii

Foreword to the First Edition xv

Preface xvii

Acknowledgements xix

Abbreviations xxi

Using this book xxiii

Introduction xxv

1 The wasted hand 01

2 Wrist drop 10

3 Proximal weakness of the arm(s) 14

4 Proximal weakness of the leg(s) 22

5 Foot drop 26

6 Ataxia and gait disturbance 33

7 Facial weakness 44

8 Ptosis 53

9 Abnormalities of vision or eye movement 58

10 Tremor and cerebellar signs 74

11 Other abnormal involuntary movements 83

12 Language and speech disturbance 97

13 Higher cortical function testing 105

14 Assessment of coma 115

15 Psychogenic (functional) neurological disorders 121

16 Telemedicine and the neurological examination 127

Picture credits 131

Index 133

List of videos

The videos listed below, and cited throughout this text, can be viewed online at www.routledge.com/ cw/morris.

Video 1	Benediction sign	05
Video 2	Deep branch lesion of the ulnar nerve	06
Video 3	Myotonic dystrophy	09
Video 4	Radial nerve lesion	10
Video 5	Inverted supinator	17
Video 6	Dressing apraxia	18
Video 7	Weakness of trapezius	19
Video 8	Weakness of serratus anterior	19
Video 9	Severe head drop	20
Video 10	Common peroneal nerve lesion	27
Video 11	Hemiparetic gait following stroke	27
Video 12	Spastic gait	35
Video 13	Motor neurone disease	35
Video 14	Antalgic gait and positive Trendelenburg sign in a patient with left sacroiliitis	37
Video 15	Gait in advanced Parkinson's disease	38
Video 16	Freezing	38
Video 17	Pull test with retropulsion in Parkinson's disease	39
Video 18	Marche à petit pas due to multiple lacunes (seen on magnetic resonance imaging (MRI))	39
Video 19	Marche à petit pas due to normal-pressure hydrocephalus	39
Video 20	Normal walking	40
Video 21	Mild cerebellar ataxia	40
Video 22	Progressive dysarthria	40
Video 23	Gait in cervical dystonia	41
Video 24	Gait in torsion dystonia	41
Video 25	Gait in Huntington's disease	41
Video 26	Dystonic camptocormia	42
Video 27	Progressive generalized dystonia	42
Video 28	Gait in dopa-induced dyskinesia	42
Video 29	Bell's palsy	44

Video 30	Hemifacial spasm	44
Video 31	Long-standing right facial palsy	46
Video 32	Left upper motor neurone facial palsy following stroke	47
Video 33	Selective right facial weakness from skin cancer	48
Video 34	Hemifacial spasm	49
Video 35	Third nerve palsy	53
Video 36	Left oculomotor (IIIrd) nerve palsy with pupillary sparing	55
Video 37	Unilateral ptosis due to myasthenia gravis	56
Video 38	Ptosis	56
Video 39	Ocular myasthenia gravis	57
Video 40	Early PSP (Steele Richardson syndrome)	62
Video 41	Left abducens (VI) nerve palsy	65
Video 42	Right trochlear (IV) nerve palsy	66
Video 43	Left internuclear ophthalmoplegia	66
Video 44	Facial and gaze palsy due to pontine metastasis	66
Video 45	Parinaud's syndrome	67
Video 46	Parinaud's syndrome	68
Video 47	Horizontal nystagmus	69
Video 48	Vertical nystagmus	70
Video 49	Horizontal pendular nystagmus	71
Video 50	Primary writing tremor	74
Video 51	Resting tremor in Parkinson's disease	75
Video 52	Resting tremor in Parkinson's disease	75
Video 53	Postural tremor in essential tremor	76
Video 54	Parkinson's disease	76
Video 55	Intention tremor	77
Video 56	Intention tremor in cerebellar disease	77
Video 57	Tremor, akinesia and gait in Parkinson's disease	77
Video 58	Falls in Parkinson's disease	78
Video 59	Speech in Parkinson's disease	78
Video 60	Holmes tremor	80
Video 61	Bat's wing tremor in a patient with Wilson's disease	81
Video 62	Slow tremor	81
Video 63	Progressive multiple system atrophy	81

Video 64	Non-fluent aphasia following intracerebral haemorrhage from a left hemisphere arteriovenous malformation (AVM)	101
Video 65	Sudden onset of mild left hemiparesis and marked left hemichorea-hemiballismus in a woman with new-onset diabetes mellitus	84
Video 66	Hemiballismus	84
Video 67	Tourette's syndrome	85
Video 68	Severe Tourette's syndrome	85
Video 69	Reflex myoclonus	86
Video 70	Post-hypoxic myoclonus	86
Video 71	Asterixis	86
Video 72	Mini-myoclonus	87
Video 73	Palatal and laryngeal myoclonus	87
Video 74	Athetosis	88
Video 75	Generalized dystonia	88
Video 76	Torticollis	88
Video 77	Craniocervical dystonia	89
Video 78	Myoclonus-dystonia syndrome	89
Video 79	Paroxysmal kinesigenic dystonia	89
Video 80	Task-specific dystonia	89
Video 81	Apraxia of eyelid opening	90
Video 82	Stereotypies	90
Video 83	Stereotypic behaviour: repeatedly pushing a button on a remote control and foot and finger tapping in a right-handed man with progressive dysarthria, apathy, anxiety and mouth drooling	90
Video 84	Dopa-induced, peak-dose dyskinesia	91
Video 85	Chorea in Huntington's disease	91
Video 86	Blepharospasm/cranial dystonia	92
Video 87	End-of-dose dystonia	93
Video 88	Tardive akathisia	94
Video 89	Akathisia	94
Video 90	Tardive dyskinesia	94
Video 91	Severe oromandibular dystonia with bruxism (constant grinding of the teeth) resulting in extensive dental damage	95
Video 92	Tardive lingual dyskinesia (stereotypy)	95
Video 93	Typical tardive dyskinesia manifested by orofacial-lingual stereotypy	95
Video 94	Tardive dystonia	96

Video 95   Wernicke's aphasia following a cardioembolic stroke   102

Video 96   Fluent aphasia in a man with a left parietal glioma   102

Video 97   Groping   107

Video 98   Frontotemporal dementia   107

Video 99   Mouth grasp   107

Video 100   Forced visual following (visual grasping)   108

Video 101   Utilization behaviour   108

Video 102   Forced mimicry   108

Video 103   Apraxia in Parkinson's disease   112

Video 104   Luria test   112

Video 105   Miming in apraxia   112

Video 106   Creutzfeldt–Jakob disease   113

Video 107   Psychogenic tics   123

Video 108   Psychogenic nystagmus and opsoclonus   125

Video 109   Psychogenic convergence spasm   125

Foreword to the Third Edition

The rites of passage from student to graduation, acceptance as a physician and then neurologist follow much the same pattern in Australia, the United Kingdom and the United States of America. Whereas in practice, the history directs physical examination, candidates in a clinical examination may be confronted with a problem as a 'short case', perhaps a single physical sign, to interpret and present a spot diagnosis or a logical approach to investigations and management. Quick thinking is aided by a mental autocue to be rolled out of our brain when required.

In the many years I have known John GL Morris, he has assiduously recorded physical signs, their history and their significance. When the affected part was stationary, he photographed it. If it moved he took a video. In this way, he has built up a collection of clinical signs that has added to his reputation as a teacher and examiner. Earlier editions of this book have proved popular as a supplement to practical work in the ward and clinic, as well as being useful as a refresher course before clinical examinations.

John GL Morris' teaming with Joseph Jankovic in presenting this new edition is a particularly happy one because of their mutual interest in movement disorders which culminated in the video collection presented here.

James W Lance, AO CBE MD FRCP FRACP FAA
*Professor Emeritus of Neurology, University of New South Wales and Honorary Consultant
Neurologist at the Prince of Wales Hospital, Sydney, Australia
Past President of the Australian Association of Neurologists (now the
Australian and New Zealand Association of Neurologists).
Fellow of the Australian Academy of Science
Past Vice President of the World Federation of Neurology
Honorary Member of the American Neurological Association and
the Association of British Neurologists
Corresponding International Member of the European Federation of Neurological Societies
Regent Member of the American Headache Society, Past President
of the International Headache Society*

Foreword to the First Edition

If medical professional life were the Grand National, the MRCP (or FRACP) would be Beecher's Brook – a daunting obstacle approached with caution, attempted with panic and surmounted with relief. Anything which makes this barrier less formidable, even to those on their third or fourth circuit of the course, is to be welcomed.

Dr Morris is a master of the old-fashioned art of clinical observation and examination and is renowned as a teacher of the subject. His wide experience as a practising clinician, instructor and examiner makes him a particularly suitable choice as an author of a book of this kind.

It is clearly written, well-illustrated and full of sensible, practical guidance, not only to those taking examinations for whom the neurology case is a particular dread but also for general physicians faced with everyday clinical problems. Even professional neurologists could scan its pages with profit and enjoyment.

Dr RW Ross Russell
Past President of the Association of British Neurologists

Preface

This little book first appeared 30 years ago as a guide to students tackling neurological 'short cases' while being observed under examination conditions. Videos were added in the second edition. In the third edition, I was joined by Joseph Jankovic, a neurologist renowned for his clinical skills, who also provided additional videos. The approach of the book was now broadened to include the neurological examination one might perform in the clinic or on a ward round. For the fourth edition, we welcome Victor Fung. I was one of the neurologists with whom Victor trained, and I have to confess that he surpassed me as a diagnostician in an indecently short time.

In an age when the emphasis on the physical examination has been eroded by increasingly sophisticated scans and other investigations, let this book be a timely reminder of the value of a well-directed neurological examination.

John Morris

Acknowledgements

John GL Morris thanks his colleagues for their help in producing *The Neurology Short Case*, out of which this book has grown: Dr Elizabeth McCusker; Professor John King; Professor Christian Lueck; Dr Rick Boyle; Dr Mariese Hely; Dr Susie Tomlinson; Professor Philip Thompson; Dr Nicholas Cordato; Professor Victor Fung (who also helped greatly with the video material); Shanthi Graham (funded in part by the Westmead Charitable Trust), who worked with him over many years on the video database and produced the video clips; Dr Roly Bigg, who through his Movement Disorder Foundation provided financial support and encouragement to build the video database; ANZAN for helping with the funding of the video database; Faith Oxley for the figures which she drew; and the following colleagues for their comments and advice on the first edition: Dr Leo Davies, Dr Jonathon Ell, Dr Ron Joffe, Dr Michael Katekar, Dr Jonathon Leicester, Dr Ivan Lorentz, Professor James McLeod, Dr Dudley O'Sullivan, Dr Ralph Ross Russell, Dr Tom Robertson, Dr Raymond Schwartz, Dr Ernest Somerville and Dr Grant Walker.

Drs Grant Walker and Jon Leicester, Professors Alasdair Corbett, Yugan Mudaliar and Richard Stark provided helpful comments on the new chapter on coma.

Professor Jankovic thanks John GL Morris for inviting him to join in the writing of this guide to the clinical examination and to contribute additional illustrative and instructive videos. These videos were selected from a library of over 30,000 videos collected at the Parkinson's Disease Center and Movement Disorders Clinic, Baylor College of Medicine, over more than three decades.

Abbreviations

ADM	abductor digiti minimi
APB	abductor pollicis brevis
A-R	Argyll Robertson
AVM	arteriovenous malformation
CT	computed tomography
DI	dorsal interosseous
ECG	electrocardiograph
EEG	electroencephalography
EMG	electromyography
ESR	erythrocyte sedimentation rate
INO	internuclear ophthalmoplegia
MND	motor neurone disease
MRA	magnetic resonance angiogram
MRI	magnetic resonance imaging
MSA	multiple system atrophy
PSP	progressive supranuclear gaze palsy
SCA	spinocerebellar ataxia
SSEPs	somatosensory evoked potentials
SSRIs	selective serotonin reuptake inhibitors

Using this book

The boxes throughout this book alert you to the free-to-access accompanying video content available online.

You can view these through your usual internet browser by going to https://www.routledge.com/cw/morris and clicking on the video of your choice, or you can access the videos directly using the QR Code.

Introduction

In this age of ever more sophisticated technology, reliance is increasingly placed on imaging, laboratory tests and electrophysiology when making a diagnosis. Inevitably, less emphasis is placed on the old-fashioned skills of history taking and clinical examination. This is even the case in neurology, where the physical examination is widely regarded as time-consuming and laborious. Yet the foundation for a sound diagnosis in neurology remains, as it always has, in the clinical assessment. The physical examination does not need to be time-consuming and laborious. The secret of the effective neurological examination lies in the ability to select those aspects of it which are relevant to each patient. Neurology is unique among the various clinical specialties in that it relies on localization of the lesion or recognition of the phenomenology before arriving at the correct diagnosis and cause. To tailor the examination successfully to the problem at hand requires a careful and detailed present, past, family and social history from the patient and this, in most cases, will take up far more time than the physical examination. The examination should have a screening component and a hypothesis-driven component. The screening component is fast and designed to pick up unexpected involvement of additional neurological systems and to allow accurate interpretation of specific signs (e.g. significant weakness will alter the interpretation of incoordination, areflexia pointing towards peripheral neuropathy which may be asymptomatic). It is often usefully performed first so that the results of a more detailed but targeted hypothesis-driven examination can be absorbed. The hypothesis-driven examination should include features expected to be abnormal if the hypothesis is correct (e.g. unsteady gait in a patient suspected of having cerebellar disease), as well as features expected to be normal if the hypothesis is correct (e.g. preserved joint position sense if the ataxia is purely from cerebellar disease). While the diagnosis is often apparent after eliciting the history, and the examination is merely confirmatory, the clinician must be familiar with and skilled in the art of examination, as this is not only an essential element of the evaluation but also engenders confidence from the patient in the thoroughness of the physician.[1]

In the chapters that follow, a simple approach to the physical examination of patients with a number of common problems will be outlined.

Technique

A brief examination can still be systematic and, as a rule, it is good to do things in the same order to lessen the chances of leaving something important out:

1. Johnston SC, Hauser SL The beautiful and ethereal neurological exam: an appeal for research. *Ann. Neurol.* 2011; 70(2): A9–A10.

● **Inspection**. You can learn a great deal by observing patients as they enter the room and while you are taking the history. Note the gait, posture, demeanour, speech, facial expression, eye movements and speech. If involuntary movements are present, note their distribution and whether they are regular in timing and rhythm (tremor), rapid and irregular (chorea, tics, myoclonus) or more sustained and patterned (the same group of muscles is always involved, as in dystonia).

● **Tone** refers to the resistance encountered in muscles when the limbs are put through a range of *passive* movements. Unfortunately, many patients try to make the doctor's task easier by actively moving their limbs during testing. Other patients resist the movements, particularly if they have not been put at ease. Active resistance against passive movement can also be seen in patients with volitional resistance in the setting of dementia ("*Gegenhalten*") or psychogenic dystonia. When testing the tone in the limbs, you should distract patients by talking to them – for example, about their social history. In order to elicit subtle arm rigidity in patients with suspected parkinsonism, ask them to repeatedly extend and flex the opposite arm at the elbow while 'feeling' for increased resistance or cogwheeling in the tested arm. A slight increase in tone occurs with this manoeuvre in normal subjects, but in Parkinson's disease, the increase may be striking and may bring out rigidity, cogwheeling or both that would not be otherwise appreciated. When testing for subtle rigidity in the legs, ask the patient to perform the repeated extension-flexion manoeuvre in the opposite arm. A useful technique in the lower limb is, with the patient lying, to roll the leg at the hip and, occasionally and without warning, to lift the knee off the bed. If the heel also lifts off the bed, tone is increased. Describe the tone as normal or increased, and if increased, whether it is velocity dependent (normal when tested with slow stretch, increased when tested with fast stretches). Hypotonia is probably not a valid term, for in a fully relaxed normal subject, no resistance is detectable to passive movement.

● **Muscle power** is tested using the techniques illustrated in *Aids to the Examination of the Peripheral Nervous System* (5th edn, WB Saunders, 2010) or *DeJong's The Neurologic Examination* (6th edn, Lippincott Williams and Wilkins, 2005). These are designed in such a way that, in most cases, you will overcome a particular muscle only if it is weak. This makes the assessment of muscle power more objective. Ensure that as far as possible, one hand of the examiner is used to stabilize the body segment(s) proximal to the joint across which the muscle tested is acting and that the other hand is not supplying resistance via pressure on a joint, which may be painful. Some muscles are more useful to test than others. Again, it is good to get into the habit of testing muscles in a certain order, as this will lessen the risk of leaving an important one out. The most useful muscles to test in the limbs are the following:
  • *Arms:* deltoid, biceps, triceps, brachioradialis, wrist extensors, finger extensors and flexors (especially flexor pollicis longus in certain clinical settings, see later), abductor pollicis brevis, abductor digiti minimi and first dorsal interosseous.

- *Legs:* gluteus maximus, iliopsoas, quadriceps, hamstrings, anterior tibial group, gastrocnemius/soleus, tibialis posterior and the peroneal muscles, toe extensors and flexors (especially extensory hallucis longus in certain clinical settings, see later).

- **Coordination**. In the upper limbs, the most sensitive way of demonstrating *cerebellar incoordination* is to get patients to try to slap their thigh alternately with the palm and back of the hand and listen to the rhythm. In cerebellar dysdiadochokinesia, the rhythm is typically irregularly irregular. The finger-to-nose test may reveal ataxia as the finger approaches the target. Akinesia associated with Parkinson's disease or other parkinsonian disorders is best tested by asking the patient to repeatedly and in rapid succession tap the thumb with the tip of the index finger, flex and extend the fingers, pronate-supinate the hands, tap the heels when the patient is seated and by repeatedly flexing-extending the hip and tapping the toes with the heels resting on the floor. In contrast to weakness, which results in persistent slowness of rapid succession movements, patients with parkinsonian akinesia have a gradually decrementing amplitude with intermittent pauses of movement (motor blocks) or even complete inability to continue a repeated movement where there is more severe bradykinesia. Lower-limb coordination is tested by getting the patient to run the heel up and down the shin (heel-to-shin manoeuvre). Finally, observing the patient during normal walking and walking in tandem is a useful way of testing leg and axial coordination. For further information on how to test patients with parkinsonism using the Unified Parkinson's Disease Rating Scale and other rating scales to assess various movement disorders, visit www.movementdisorders.org/publications/rating_scales/.

- Be careful how you interpret incoordination in a patient in whom you have demonstrated muscle weakness. Patients with weak muscles find tests of coordination difficult to perform. As a rule, it is better to assume that incoordination in the presence of muscle weakness sufficient to impair anti-gravity movements is due to that cause. Loss of proprioception may also cause incoordination.

- **Reflexes**, deep tendon, cutaneous and nociceptive are crucial in determining the likely location of a lesion and the diagnosis. It is often difficult to elicit ankle jerks in the elderly due to poor relaxation. Do not accept that a reflex is absent until you have tapped the Achilles tendon with the patient kneeling on a chair and done the Jendrassik reinforcement. For the upper-limb reflexes, get the patient to make a fist with the other hand or clench the teeth; for the lower-limb reflexes, ask the patient to hook their hands together in a monkey grip and to try to pull them apart on command. The manoeuvre is most effective if the tendon is tapped immediately after the command to pull. In addition to the deep tendon reflexes, it is also important to try to elicit the Babinski sign or the extensor plantar response. When present, as evidenced by extension and fanning of the toes in response to *nociceptive* stimulation of the lateral aspect of the sole of the foot, the Babinski sign provides evidence for a lesion in the corticospinal or pyramidal tract. As some patients are unusually sensitive (ticklish) and have a nonspecific withdrawal response, it is helpful to use other supportive signs of corticospinal or pyramidal tract involvement. These include toe-extension signs, such as the Chaddock sign (elicited by stimulating the lateral aspect of the foot), Oppenheim sign (elicited by applying pressure to the anterior aspect of the tibia) or the Gordon sign (elicited by applying deep pressure to the calf muscles). In contrast, the Rossolimo sign (elicited by tapping the ball of the foot) and the Mendel-Bechterew sign (elicited by stroking the lateral aspect of the dorsum of the foot) result in a slightly delayed, quick plantar flexion of the toes in patients with pyramidal tract lesions.

- **Sensory testing** is the least reliable aspect of the examination, and in most cases, it is not something on which to spend a great time of time. Minor differences in sensation between different parts of the body are common and are usually of no significance. Perception of sensation is also affected by whether the part of the body being tested is painful or weak. Many patients with, for example, Bell's palsy or trigeminal neuralgia (disorders not usually associated with sensory loss) will say that the skin on the affected side feels different. In general, the sensory examination should be performed towards the end of the neurological examination and be especially hypothesis-driven (e.g. differentiating between a dermatomal versus peripheral nerve distribution of sensory loss in a patient with a C8 versus ulnar nerve lesion).

- Always examine both spinothalamic and dorsal column modalities, which may be preferentially affected in dissociated or crossed sensory impairment. Temperature sensation is more sensitive and pinprick more specific for spinothalamic sensory loss, vibration sense more sensitive and joint position sense more specific for dorsal column sensory loss. Light touch is carried by both pathways. More weight is given to a sensory disturbance if perception of a particular modality appears to be lost rather than altered. Ask the patient to say 'yes' each time the skin is lightly touched (with the eyes shut) and to distinguish between the blunt and sharp ends of a disposable pin applied repeatedly to an area of skin. In testing vibration, confirm that patients really can feel the sensation by asking them when it stops. After a suitable pause, terminate the vibration by touching the end of the tuning fork.

- There are certain circumstances in which you must make time to assess sensation:
  - In a patient with absent ankle jerks and bladder symptoms (suggesting a lesion of the cauda equina), it is essential to test sensation in the lower limbs and particularly in the perineal regions that are supplied by the lower sacral dermatomes.
  - In a patient with paraparesis, you must look for a sensory level. If there is impaired sensation in the legs, establish the level at which this occurs, moving the stimulus

(pin [pain] or finger [touch]) repeatedly from the numb to the normal area. Test the front and back of the limbs and trunk. It is often useful to move a vibrating tuning fork (128 Hz) one segment at a time up the vertebral spines or to drag the base up the legs and trunk and determine where it begins to feel cold. Cause the tuning fork to vibrate by plucking it between thumb and index finger. Banging it on the bed causes audible vibration and invalidates the test.

- In a patient with suspected motor neurone disease, it is essential to show that sensation is normal.

- **Screening tests**. These are carried out in a few moments and allow you to narrow down on a particular part or system for more detailed examination:

  - *Face*. Make a point of observing the patient's facial expressions as you take the history. Listen to their voice. If cerebral imaging has not been recently performed, fundoscopy should be performed in all patients to detect unexpected raised intracranial pressure from a space-occupying lesion. Testing with simultaneous finger movements in the left and right upper-outer and then lower-outer quadrants will detect almost all major unexpected visual field deficits (isolated binasal hemianopia is extremely rare). Test for conjugate saccadic and pursuit eye movements, looking for nystagmus at the extremes of horizontal and vertical gaze. Ptosis will be obvious during this examination. Look particularly for facial asymmetry or loss of expression. Examine palatal elevation while at the same time looking at the tongue for gross wasting or fasciculation. Check for craniotomy scars and note any unexpected baldness.

  - *Arms*. Ask patients to put their arms out in front of them in the pronated position, to hold their arms there for a few moments with the eyes shut looking for arm drift and then to touch their nose with each index finger in turn. Screen for gross weakness by asking the patient to push the whole arm while still pronated up from the horizontal while applying resistance with your fingers perpendicularly placed on the dorsal aspect of their fingers. This is a reasonably sensitive *screening* test for detecting unsuspected pyramidal weakness (that affected shoulder abduction > adduction and finger extension > flexion), as well as proximal (deltoid) weakness from myopathy or distal (finger extension) weakness from neuropathy. These simple manoeuvres will often reveal important clues such as weakness, sensory loss, intention tremor, postural tremor, wrist drop and dystonia.

  - *Legs*. Get the patient to walk in an open space. Observe the posture, arm swing and stride. Note whether the patient walks on a wide base or whether there is unsteadiness on turning. Ask the patient to walk in tandem (heel to toe). If neuromuscular disease is suspected, ask them to rise from a squatting position (testing proximal power) and to stand on their toes and heels (testing distal power). You should also test balance using the *Romberg's sign* and the *pull test* (see the following).

● **Formulation of a diagnosis**. By the time you have finished the examination you should have come to some conclusions on at least two key questions: *'Where is the lesion?'*, and/or *'What is the phenomenology?'* Occasionally, the patient will have pathognomonic signs that allow you to also reasonably answer the question *'What is the likely underlying cause?'*, but more often, the etiological differential diagnosis also relies on important components of the history, especially the *temporal course* of the illness, *intercurrent illness or comorbidity, medication or drug exposure* and *any family history*. In the letter which you write to the referring doctor, you need to commit yourself to making a diagnosis with, in some cases, a short differential diagnosis. *Don't be a doctor who lists every possible cause and test, for fear of being wrong. That helps no one. If you prove to be wrong, then you will have learned something.* Certain patterns of signs are useful in determining the site of the lesion:

- Generalized distal weakness is likely to be due to a peripheral neuropathy. Generalized proximal weakness is likely to be due to a myopathy.
- If a muscle is weak due to a peripheral nerve lesion, then all muscles innervated by that nerve below the site of the lesion will also be weak. For example, if brachioradialis is weak due to a lesion of the radial nerve in the spiral groove of the humerus, then extension of the fingers and wrist must also be weak. If they are not, then the problem must be elsewhere.
- In the case of an upper motor neurone disorder of the leg, the lesion must be above the level of the second lumbar vertebra. Whether the lesion is in the cord or above is determined by examining the upper limbs and cranial nerves.
- If you have decided that the signs suggest a lower motor neurone disorder, it is helpful to consider whether the lesion is likely to be in the anterior horn cell, root, plexus, peripheral nerve, neuromuscular junction or muscle.
- In a cord lesion, reflexes are lost at the level of the lesion and increased below the lesion.
- In a unilateral brainstem lesion above the medulla, there may be 'crossed' signs with a cranial nerve lesion ipsilateral to the lesion and hemiparesis contralateral to the lesion.

As students, we were drawn to neurology by the ability of our teachers to make a diagnosis relying almost entirely on their clinical skills. The neurological examination when conducted by a master of the art is a beautiful if not ethereal experience. We hope that through using the approaches outlined in the chapters ahead that your neurological examination will go some way to reaching that ideal.

1 The wasted hand

Inspection 01
Distribution of wasting 02
Power, coordination and reflexes 03

This is usually a chronic condition and patients present with weakness of the hand(s) or numbness/tingling. They may have noticed muscle wasting.

The small muscles of the hand are supplied by the median and ulnar nerves and the C8/T1 roots. In a root lesion, usually both median and ulnar innervated muscles are affected; in a single peripheral nerve lesion, wasting is selective.

Inspection

Upon noting wasting of the small muscles of the hand, check the following:

- **The patient's age**. Some loss of muscle bulk is normal in the elderly, but this is symmetrical in the two hands, and the wasted muscles are not weak.

- **Arthritis**. This also causes wasting with minimal weakness (allowing for the pain which testing power may induce). Subluxation of the metacarpal bone of the thumb causes selective wasting of the thenar eminence, which may be mistaken for a median nerve lesion. Patients with Parkinson's disease and other causes of parkinsonism often manifest 'striatal deformities' of the hands and feet, which may be wrongly attributed to arthritis. The typical striatal hand deformity consists of flexion of the metacarpophalangeal joints, extension of the proximal interphalangeal joints and flexion of the distal interphalangeal joints without evidence of joint swelling or tenderness (see Figure 1.1), although some fixed deformity of the joint can develop if long-standing.

- **Pupils**. A smaller pupil with ptosis, with lowering of the upper eyelid and elevation of the lower eyelid due to weakness of Müller's orbital muscle (Horner's syndrome)[1] and a wasted hand suggests a C8/T1 root or cord lesion. Inequality of the pupils due to Horner's syndrome is most obvious in a dimly lit room.

1. Johann Friedrich Horner, Swiss ophthalmologist (1831–1886).

DOI: 10.1201/9781003119166-1

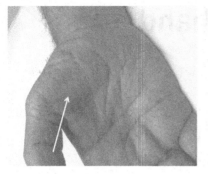
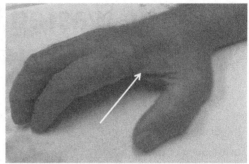

Wasting of thenar eminence   Wasting of FDI

Figure 1.1 **Split hand in motor neuron disease.**

Note disproportionate wasting of abductor pollicis brevis (APB) and opponens pollicis (thenar eminence) and first dorsal interosseous (DI) muscles with relative preservation of the adductor digiti minimi (ADM; hypothenar eminence). (Figure courtesy of Steve Vucic & Parvathi Menon).

Because sympathetic innervation and the medial longitudinal fasciculus extend caudally to the lower cervical and upper thoracic areas, Horner's syndrome and internuclear ophthalmoplegia (INO) are two neuro-ophthalmological signs which may accompany lesions in these anatomical areas.

- **Clawing** of the ring and little fingers (due to weakness of the lumbrical muscles) suggests an ulnar nerve lesion.

- **Fasciculations** suggest motor neurone disease (MND).

- **Length of the two hands** and the size of the thumbnails. Hemiatrophy (more accurately hemi-smallness, as it reflects failure of growth rather than wasting) suggests injury to the nervous system in infancy (polio, birth trauma, stroke).

- **Scars** in the arms, especially over the elbow (ulnar nerve trauma).

Distribution of wasting

Take particular note of three muscles: ADM, first DI (1st DI) and APB (see Figures 1.2 and 1.3). There are three common patterns of wasting:

- *Wasting confined to APB.* Usually a median nerve lesion. Rarely due to cervical rib.

- *Wasting confined to ADM and 1st DI.* The patient has an ulnar nerve lesion.

- *Wasting of all three muscles.* Several possibilities (see the following).

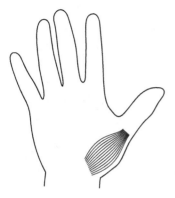

Figure 1.2 APB.

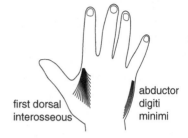

first dorsal interosseous

abductor digiti minimi

Figure 1.3 1st DI and ADM.

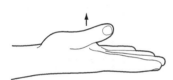

Figure 1.4 Abduction of the thumb.

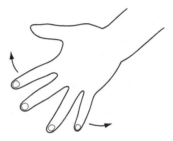

Figure 1.5 Abduction of the fingers.

Power, coordination and reflexes

After the arm raising screening test, test power in the deltoid, biceps, triceps, brachioradialis, wrist extensors, finger extensors and then APB, ADM and 1st DI (Figures 1.4 and 1.5). Test coordination and all the reflexes in the upper limbs. There are three common patterns of weakness:

- Weakness confined to APB is usually due to entrapment of the median nerve at the wrist within the carpal tunnel. If it is due to a lesion at the elbow, there will also be weakness of the deep flexors of the index finger and of the flexor pollicis longus (Figure 1.6). Ask the patient to make a fist; he or she may have the 'Benediction sign'[2] (Figure 1.7a). Test power in the terminal phalanges of the index and thumb by getting the patient to form a figure 'O' with those digits (Figure 1.7b). If those muscles are weak, the digits will assume the posture shown in Figure 1.7c. In more subtle weakness, it is necessary to test flexor pollicis and/or the digit 2 flexor digitorum profundus individually. Flexor pollicis is a powerful muscle – if the patient is asked to flex the interphalangeal joint of the thumb at a right angle, it

2. Confusingly, the Benediction sign is also sometimes used to describe the posture in an ulnar nerve lesion where there is clawing of the ring and little fingers; in an ulnar nerve lesion, the 'Benediction' posture is seen at rest in a median nerve lesion on attempting to make a fist.

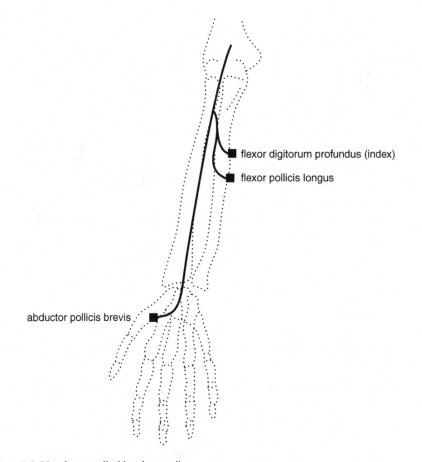

flexor digitorum profundus (index)

flexor pollicis longus

abductor pollicis brevis

Figure 1.6 Muscles supplied by the median nerve.

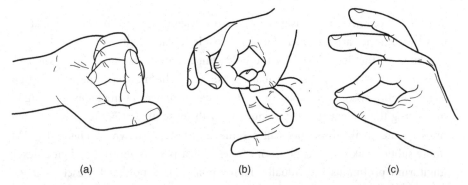

(a)   (b)   (c)

Figure 1.7 (a) Benediction sign of a proximal lesion of the median nerve, (b) testing flexor pollicis longus and the deep flexor of the index and (c) posture adopted when flexor pollicis longus and the deep flexor of the index are weak.

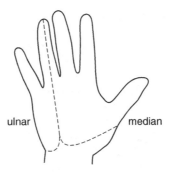

Figure 1.8 Sensory distribution of the median and ulnar nerves.

should not be possible to pull it straight using the tip of the examiner's index finger unless it is weak. Test the digit 2–5 deep finger flexors by seeing whether you can use your own index finger to pry their fingertips off while they are strongly gripping an ophthalmoscope handle. *When faced with wasting of the thenar eminence and/or weakness of APB, weakness of flexor pollicis brevis places the level of the lesion above the level of the wrist, most commonly at a proximal median or lower trunk/medial cord of brachial plexus level.* Test whether there is a sensory loss in the distribution of the median nerve (Figure 1.8).

See Video 1 Benediction sign

The patient fails to flex the terminal phalanx of the thumb and index. There is wasting of the thenar eminence. The patient has a proximal median nerve lesion.

● Weakness confined to ADM and 1st DI is usually due to an ulnar nerve lesion at the elbow (see Figure 1.9). In severe cases, there will also be weakness of the deep flexor of the little finger (see Figure 1.10). Ensure that APB (taking care to test power strictly in the thumb abduction plane) and finger extension are unaffected, to exclude more proximal C8/T1 pathology as the cause, of the weakness. Test for sensory loss in an ulnar distribution (Figure 1.8).

In the rare lesion of the deep palmar branch of the ulnar nerve, weakness is confined to abduction of the index, and there is no sensory loss.

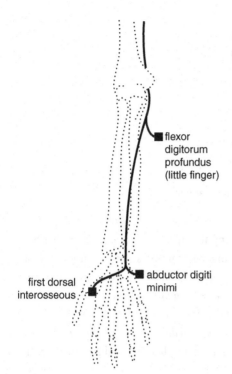

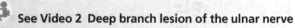

Figure 1.9 Muscles supplied by the ulnar nerve.

Figure 1.10 Weakness of flexor digito-rum profundus of the little finger (proximal lesion of the ulnar nerve).

See Video 2 Deep branch lesion of the ulnar nerve
The patient is unable to abduct the index finger on the right, and there is wasting of the 1st DI muscle.

- Weakness of all three muscles has many causes, and it is not possible to make a definite diagnosis without performing a full neurological examination. In particular, it is important to check for the following:
  - Horner's syndrome
  - ptosis
  - facial weakness
  - wasting of the tongue
  - jaw jerk
  - wasting of the sternomastoids
  - wasting, weakness and reflex changes in all four limbs
  - sensory loss

Probably the most common cause of weakness of all three muscles is a combined median neuropathy at the wrist and ulnar neuropathy at the elbow, as both are common entrapment neuropathies. Co-morbid diabetes mellitus is a common risk factor that predisposes to severe focal compressive neuropathy of both the median and ulnar nerves but is not invariably present. Sensory loss should be limited to the median and ulnar nerve distributions, and not extend above the wrist.

Certain patterns of neurological signs associated with wasting of the small muscles of the hand are characteristic of the following:

● Wasting confined to one hand and weakness of the finger extensors, finger flexors and triceps. The triceps reflex is absent, and there is sensory loss on the ulnar aspect of the forearm and hand (see Figure 1.11). The patient has a C7, C8, T1 root or plexus lesion. If this is due to a cervical rib, there may also be a subclavian bruit and diminished pulses in the arm. In a Pancoast tumour, there may be a Horner's syndrome, bovine cough, signs in the chest, lymphadenopathy and cachexia.

● 'Flail' arm with flaccid paralysis, wasting, areflexia and sensory loss confined to one arm. The most common cause of this is avulsion of all the roots of the brachial plexus from C5-T1, often resulting from a motorbike accident. Look for evidence of more proximal C5 myotomal involvement with wasting and weakness of shoulder girdle muscles such as supraspinatus (weakness of the first 30 degrees of shoulder abduction) and serratus anterior (winging of the scapula). Horner's syndrome is usually present.

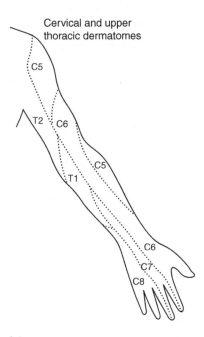

Figure 1.11 Dermatomes of the arm.

- Wasting of one hand, loss of reflexes in the arm and a dissociated sensory loss (loss of pain with preserved touch sensation) in a half-cape distribution on the same side. The hands may be swollen, cold and blue with the skin shiny, atrophic and scarred from previous unnoticed injuries. These are signs of an intrinsic lesion of the cervical and upper thoracic cord. Syringomyelia and tumours, such as ependymoma, should be considered. The signs may be bilateral.

- Wasting of both hands and spastic weakness of the legs. The patient has a C8,T1 cord lesion. There will usually be sensory loss to the appropriate level. Causes of this include tumour and trauma.

- Generalized muscle weakness and wasting, fasciculations, hyperreflexia and normal sensation. The patient has MND. Check the tongue for wasting and fasciculations. A characteristic pattern of wasting and weakness occurs in almost all patients with motor neuron disease, known as the 'split hand'. APB and flexor digitorum indicis (FDI) are more severely affected than ADM [VF NEW FIG 1.1]. This is hypothesized to be due to greater cortical representation of the thumb and index finger muscles that are important in a pincer grip, making them more vulnerable to the cortically driven component of neurodegeneration in MND.

- Distal wasting and weakness of all four limbs, areflexia and a glove and stocking sensory loss. The patient has a peripheral neuropathy.

- Distal wasting and weakness of all four limbs, hyporeflexia, baldness, ptosis and cataracts. Cognitive slowing, drowsiness and the presence of a cardiac monitor or permanent pacemaker are other clues. The patient probably has dystrophia myotonica. Ask them to make a tight fist and then to open the fingers as rapidly as possible. If the fingers unfurl slowly, they have myotonia. Tap the thenar eminence. If the thumb slowly abducts and then falls back to its original position, they also have percussion myotonia.

- Rarely, weakness isolated to the intrinsic hand muscles in the absence of upper motor neurone signs can develop as a consequence of focal, localized pathology of the hand area of the primary motor cortex. Look for clumsiness and inability to fractionate finger movements (sequentially touching the tips of each of digits 2–5 to the tip of the thumb) that is disproportionate to the degree of weakness (which is shown to be minor by demonstrating that the patient can easily flex and extend all the fingers at once when opening and closing a fist).

 See Video 3: Myotonic dystrophy

Frontal baldness, ptosis, failure to bury the eyelashes, myotonia causing slowing of fist opening and percussion myotonia of thumb adduction.

Box 1.1	Tips

- Cervical spondylosis is very common in older patients, but, in most cases, it is *not* the cause of marked muscle wasting in the hand; other causes should be considered.

- Generalized fasciculations are a key sign in the diagnosis of MND. If you are considering this diagnosis, it is essential to disrobe the patient and to make a point of observing all parts of the musculature. Fasciculation is best seen by fixing the foveal gaze on the mid-part of the limb segment of interest and using peripheral vision, which is more sensitive to movement to pick up the subtle muscle twitch. Fasciculation is often best seen in triceps, the wrist extensors and FDI. Flickering movements of the calves and of the protruded tongue are common in normal individuals. Fasciculations in a relaxed tongue, however, may suggest denervation. They may also be seen in a generalized distribution in normal individuals. As a rule, fasciculation is rarely a matter of concern in the absence of weakness or muscle wasting.

- The most common cause of coldness in a wasted hand is not vascular occlusion, but disuse.

- The most common causes of wasting of the small muscles of the hands are old age and arthritis; in these conditions, muscle power in the wasted muscles is preserved.

2 Wrist drop

Inspection 10
Tone 11
Power, coordination and reflexes 12

This is usually an acute phenomenon following compression of the radial nerve in the spiral groove of the humerus after falling asleep in a chair ('Saturday night palsy'). The nerve may also suffer infarction due to occlusion of the vasa nervorum in diabetes mellitus. Wrist extension is also weak in corticospinal lesions.

Wrist drop is due to weakness of extensor carpi radialis longus (supplied by C5/6 and the radial nerve) and extensor carpi ulnaris (supplied by C7/8 and the posterior interosseous branch of the radial nerve). It most commonly results from compression of the radial nerve in the spiral groove (Figure 2.1).

See Video 4 Radial nerve lesion
Wrist drop on the right, failure to abduct the fingers in the flexed posture, failure to contract brachioradialis on wrist flexion against resistance.

Inspection

Wrist drop is seen when the arms are held out during the screening examination. In a posterior interosseous nerve lesion or C7/8 root lesion, there will be radial deviation of the hand because of sparing of extensor carpi radialis longus (Figure 2.1). In a corticospinal lesion, the arm is slow to elevate and the elbow and wrist may remain a little flexed. Check for

● bruising or scars, particularly over the spiral groove of the humerus in the posterior part of the upper arm (radial nerve palsy);

DOI: 10.1201/9781003119166-2

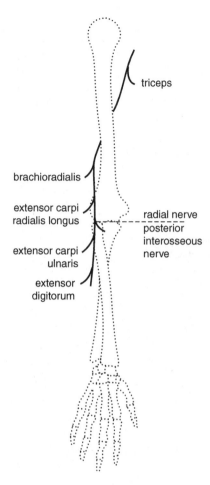

Figure 2.1 Muscles supplied by the radial nerve.

- facial asymmetry (hemiparesis); and/or

- muscle wasting, particularly in the extensor compartment of the forearm. Allow for the fact that the right forearm is usually thicker than the left in a right-handed person.

Tone

Tone in the upper limbs will be normal in a lesion of the peripheral nerve or roots and usually increased in a corticospinal lesion.

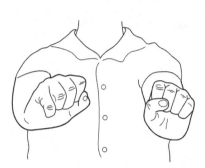

Figure 2.2 Radial deviation in wrist drop due to a posterior interosseous nerve lesion.

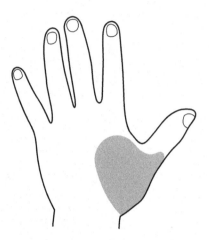

Figure 2.3 Sensory loss over the snuff box in a radial nerve lesion.

Power, coordination and reflexes

Test shoulder abduction, elbow flexion, elbow extension, brachioradialis, wrist extension, finger extension, finger flexion, finger abduction and thumb abduction. Test finger abduction with the hand and wrist firmly supported such as resting on a hard surface (see Tips). Check coordination and reflexes in the upper limbs.

You are likely to find one of four patterns of weakness:

- Weakness of brachioradialis, wrist extension and finger extension. The patient has a radial nerve lesion. As triceps is normal and brachioradialis is weak, the lesion is likely to be in the spiral groove. The brachioradialis reflex is reduced or absent. There may be sensory loss in the region of the snuff box (Figure 2.3).

- Weakness of finger extension with radial deviation of the wrist on attempted extension, signifying weakness of extensor carpi ulnaris (Figure 2.2). There is no sensory loss, and reflexes are normal. The patient has a posterior interosseous nerve lesion (rare). This may result from entrapment of the nerve or be part of a mononeuritis multiplex (or simplex) of any cause (e.g. diabetes, collagen disease).

- Weakness of triceps and finger extensors and flexors; radial deviation of the wrist on attempted extension. The triceps reflex is reduced or absent. The patient has a C7/8 root or plexus lesion. These signs may be seen in cervical spondylosis or a brachial plexus injury.

- Generalized weakness of the muscles of the upper limb which is most marked in deltoid, triceps, wrist extension and finger extension. The patient has a corticospinal lesion. Tone and reflexes are likely to be increased. Look for weakness in the face and leg on the same side (hemiparesis).

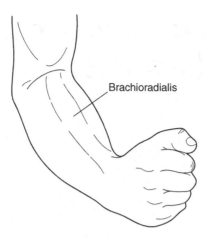

Brachioradialis

Figure 2.4 Brachioradialis.

Box 2.1   Tips

● It is almost impossible to abduct the fingers when they are flexed at the metocarpophalangeal joints. Try it yourself. In wrist drop, the fingers are also flexed and it is essential, therefore, for you to correct this before asking the patient to attempt to perform finger abduction. This is best done by firmly supporting the hand and wrist in the prone position on a hard flat surface.

● Brachioradialis is the key muscle to test in a suspected radial nerve palsy (Figure 2.4).

3 Proximal weakness of the arm(s)

Inspection 15
Tone 16
Power, coordination and reflexes 16

Here the patient may complain of difficulty putting clothes on the line or holding the arm up to use a screwdriver. The differential diagnosis very much depends on whether one arm or both are affected (see the following).

The proximal muscles of the upper limb which are routinely tested are

- deltoid: shoulder abduction; axillary nerve; C5/6 roots;

- biceps: elbow flexion; musculocutaneous nerve; C5/6 roots;

- triceps: elbow extension; radial nerve; C7/8 roots; and

- brachioradialis: elbow flexion with the thumb pointing to the nose; radial nerve; C5/6 roots.

Under some circumstances, it is useful to test

- supraspinatus: first 20° of shoulder abduction; suprascapular nerve; C5/6 roots;

- infraspinatus: external rotation at the shoulder; suprascapular nerve; C5/6 roots;

- trapezius: shoulder elevation; spinal accessory nerve (superior portion); C3/4 (inferior portion); and

- serratus anterior: scapular fixation and rotation; long thoracic nerve; C5/6/7.

The deltoid can only function effectively if the scapula is firmly anchored by trapezius and serratus anterior (Figure 3.1). Rotation of the scapula increases the range of abduction possible at the shoulder.

Unilateral weakness confined to the proximal upper limb is usually due to a lesion of the cervical roots, brachial plexus or peripheral nerves. In corticospinal lesions, all the

DOI: 10.1201/9781003119166-3

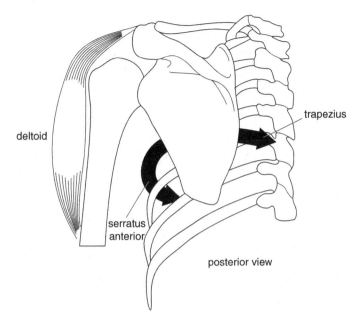

Figure 3.1 Mode of action of trapezius and serratus anterior on the scapula.

extensors of the upper limb, proximal and distal, are weak. Bilateral proximal weakness of the upper limbs raises the possibility of a myopathy.

Inspection

Remove all garments from the patient's trunk and upper limbs and look for the following:

- **Skin**. A purple ('heliotrope') rash around the eyes and on the cheeks and a scaly erythema at the base of the fingernails and on the elbows and knees are features of dermatomyositis.

- **Joints**. Look for subluxation of the humerus (Figure 3.2).

- **Wasting**. This is most obvious in the deltoid. Look at the shoulder from the back as well as the front or you may miss winging of the scapula. Look also for wasting of other shoulder girdle muscles, especially supraspinatus and trapezius.

- **Face**. This may provide important clues: unilateral ptosis (Horner's syndrome with an avulsion injury of the cervical roots and T1), bilateral ptosis (dystrophica myotonia, myasthenia gravis, myopathy), facial droop (as part of a hemiparesis).

- **Fasciculation**. MND.

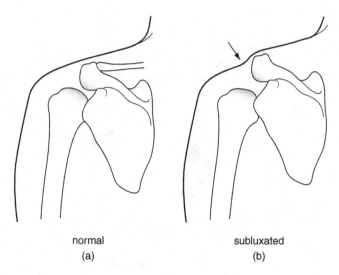

normal
(a)

subluxated
(b)

Figure 3.2 (a) Profile of normal shoulder joint; (b) profile of shoulder in downward subluxation of the humerus.

Tone

This will be normal in disorders of the peripheral nerves or muscle and may be increased in a corticospinal lesion.

Power, coordination and reflexes

Test shoulder abduction, elbow flexion and extension, brachioradialis, wrist extension and flexion and finger extension, flexion and abduction. Check coordination and reflexes in the upper limbs. There are a number of characteristic patterns of weakness, each associated with other signs:

● Weakness confined to the deltoid. This cannot be a C5/6 root lesion for biceps, and brachioradialis is spared (Figure 3.3). Make certain that the scapula does not move as the arm gives way when shoulder abduction is tested. If it does not, the patient has an axillary nerve lesion. Reflexes will be normal. There may be an area of sensory loss over the deltoid.

● Weakness of deltoid, biceps and brachioradialis, with normal power in the other muscles tested so far. This is a C5/6 cord, root or plexus lesion. To determine the level of the lesion, other signs need to be considered:

   • C5/6 cord lesion. Here, the reflexes at the level of the lesion – biceps and brachioradialis – are depressed, while those below that level – triceps and the lower

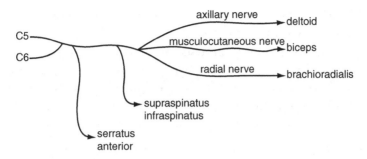

Figure 3.3 Muscles supplied by C5 and C6.

limb reflexes – are increased. The vibration caused by tapping the radius to elicit the brachioradialis reflex may cause the fingers to flex; the finger flexors arise below the site of the lesion (at C7/8) and are therefore more easily excited. Some flexion is common in normal individuals, but if flexion of the fingers occurs without contraction of the brachioradialis in response to tapping of the radius (the 'inverted supinator' reflex), a C5/6 cord lesion is probably present. Test tone and power in the lower limbs and look for a sensory level at C5.

 See Video 5 Inverted supinator
The fingers flex when the radius is tapped, but there is no reflex contraction in brachioradialis. The triceps jerk is brisk.

- C5/6 root or plexus lesion. Here, the biceps and brachioradialis reflexes are absent, but the triceps reflex and leg reflexes are normal. The point at which these nerves have been damaged is determined by testing muscles, also supplied by the C5/6 roots in the order in which they arise (Figure 3.3). Thus, a very proximal lesion will involve all the C5/6 muscles. Further down, serratus anterior is spared and further down still, supraspinatus and infraspinatus will be spared. In a C5/6 root or plexus lesion, there is likely to be sensory loss in the same dermatomes (see Figure 1.10).

● Weakness of all the muscles of one arm with the following:
- Absence of reflexes in the arm. If the other limbs are normal, the patient probably has a brachial plexus lesion. Check for a Horner's syndrome and a

C5-T1 sensory loss. If there is a dissociated sensory loss, consider intrinsic cord lesions such as syringomyelia.

- Hyperreflexia. Use your screening tests on the face and legs to determine whether this is part of a hemiparesis. With a right hemiparesis, check for aphasia (see the following). With a left hemiparesis, test for signs of neglect (sensory and visual), constructional apraxia and dressing apraxia.

 See Video 6 Dressing apraxia
The patient gets into a tangle trying to put her jacket back on, having inadvertently pulled the left sleeve inside out.

- Weakness of the proximal muscles of both arms. This is likely to be due to a disorder of muscle (myopathy) or neuromuscular junction. Test power and reflexes in the lower limbs. There are several characteristic patterns of signs:
  - Weakness of all the proximal muscles of the arms and legs. Reflexes are normal or reduced. Sensation is normal. Consider polymyositis, particularly in an older person, if there is muscle tenderness on palpation or if there is a skin rash (dermatomyositis). Myasthenia gravis is also a possibility. Check for fatigability by asking the patient to do 20 repetitions of wing beats on one side, and retest strength bilaterally to see if there is excessive fatigue, evidenced by marked asymmetry in resistance that is unmasked by the exercise. Test for weakness of neck flexion (see Box 3.1). Look for progressive ptosis with prolonged upgaze (which make take 30–60 s to develop).
  - Selective weakness and wasting of the proximal muscles of the arms and legs. Here, certain muscles are almost completely wasted while their neighbour, perhaps with the same root supply, is normal. Thus, brachioradialis (C5/6) may be wasted while deltoid (also C5/6) is spared. There may be winging of the scapula. These are the findings of muscular dystrophy, spinal muscular atrophy and inclusion body myositis. Test facial movements and eye closure. The patient could be of any age but is more likely to be young. If the reflexes are lost, you should consider spinal muscular atrophy.

● Weakness of the muscles which fixate the scapula usually becomes apparent during testing of the deltoid. You find weakness of shoulder abduction, but on careful inspection and palpation, it becomes clear that you are not 'breaking' the deltoid, rather you are forcing the scapula to rotate. The patient has weakness of the trapezius, serratus anterior or both. Check the following:

- Note the position of the shoulders. In weakness of the trapezius, one shoulder will be lower than the other. Compare the muscle bulk of the trapezius on the two sides. Wasting of the trapezius is often visible and palpable.

 See Video 7 Weakness of trapezius

The right shoulder is depressed; there is limitation of abduction of the right shoulder; the right scapula wings when the arms are pushed against the wall.

- Compare the sternocleidomastoids on both sides. Ask the patient to turn their head to either side and press their cheek against your hand. This will allow easy palpation of the sternocleidomastoid muscle and observation for hypotrophy, as seen in patients with dystonic torticollis, or atrophy, present with lesions of the accessory nerve. The accessory nerve supplies both trapezius and sternocleidomatoid.
- Ask the patient to push the extended arms against the wall. The vertebral border of the scapula lifts away from the thorax ('wings') if there is weakness of the serratus anterior. Isolated weakness of the serratus anterior is quite common. It follows injury to the long thoracic nerve by, for example, cervical gland biopsy. It is also one manifestation of neuralgic amyotrophy (brachial neuritis).

 See Video 8 Weakness of serratus anterior

The right scapula lifts away from the chest wall when the arms are extended at the shoulder.

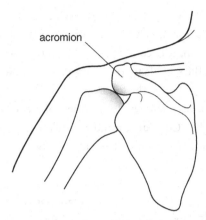

acromion

Figure 3.4 Restriction of abduction of the humerus by the acromion in upward subluxation associated with a rotator cuff tear.

Box 3.1   Tips

- Weakness of shoulder abduction can be due to weakness of the deltoid or failure of serratus anterior and trapezius to fixate the scapula. Feel the tip of the scapula with one hand as you test shoulder abduction with the other hand. If the scapula moves, the problem is at least in part due to weakness of the serratus anterior or trapezius. The strength of the deltoid can be tested separately by manually fixating the scapula as you test shoulder abduction.

- Brachioradialis is one of the most useful muscles to test. It is important in diagnosing C5/6 root lesions and in localizing the site of a radial nerve lesion. It is often selectively wasted in muscular dystrophy. Both biceps and brachioradialis flex the elbow; weakness of brachioradialis cannot be demonstrated by overcoming elbow flexion, for biceps is more than adequate for this task. Weakness in brachioradialis is detected by observing and feeling the muscle when elbow flexion is resisted with the forearm midway between pronation and supination (see Figure 2.5): 'Pull your thumb towards your nose'. A weak brachioradialis remains soft during this procedure or fails to contract at all.

- Always test for weakness of neck flexion or extension when you find proximal weakness of the arms. This is characteristically present in myopathies and myasthenia gravis.

 See Video 9 Severe head drop

Occurred as a result of neck extensor weakness due to acetylcholine receptor antibody-positive myasthenia gravis.

- Rotator cuff injuries to the shoulder can be confusing. When asked to abduct the shoulder, they are only able to do so to a limited extent, and you may mistakenly diagnose an axillary nerve lesion. The following features should make you consider this possibility:

    - Abduction against resistance is usually painful. The range of passive movement of the shoulder is limited and also elicits pain when examined.

    - While abduction is limited, forward flexion of the elbow is normal. The reason for this is that the humerus subluxates upwards when the rotator cuff is ruptured and the coracoid bone prevents full abduction (Figure 3.4).

    - The long head of biceps is ruptured, causing the biceps to 'bunch up' in elbow flexion.

    - On attempted abduction, the shoulder is elevated, giving it a characteristic shrugging appearance.

4 Proximal weakness of the leg(s)

Inspection 22

Tone 23

Power, coordination and reflexes 23

With proximal weakness of the lower limbs, the patient has difficulty getting out of a chair or climbing the stairs. Walking may also be affected.

The proximal muscles of the legs which are routinely tested are as follows:

● Iliopsoas: hip flexion; femoral nerve; L1/2/3 roots

● Quadriceps: knee extension; femoral nerve; L2/3/4 roots

● Gluteus maximus: hip extension; inferior gluteal nerve; L5, S1/2 roots

● Hamstrings: knee flexion; sciatic nerve; L5, S1/2 roots

● Hip adductors: obturator nerve; L2/3/4

Weakness which is confined to the proximal muscles of the legs is usually due to a disorder of muscle (e.g. myopathy) or neuromuscular junction (e.g. myasthenia gravis). Weakness of proximal and distal muscles is seen in Guillain-Barré[1] syndrome and MND. Unilateral proximal weakness is often due to a femoral nerve lesion.

Inspection

Observe the gait. This may include

● waddling, with exaggerated shoulder sway, in any cause of proximal weakness or in hip joint disorders;

● antalgic, the stride when weight bearing on the painful side is faster and shorter than on the good side; or

● hemiparetic (see section on gait).

1. Georges Guillain, French neurologist at the Salpetriere, Paris (1876–1961); JA Barré, French neurologist (1880–1967).

DOI: 10.1201/9781003119166-4

Ask the patient to rise from a crouching position. Patients with proximal weakness of the lower limbs cannot get up. Children with muscular dystrophy may 'climb up' themselves, using their arms as levers (Gowers'[2] sign).

- Look for wasting in quadriceps. This is most obvious with the patient standing. You may wish to compare the circumference of the thighs at a defined distance above the knee, but it is difficult to do this accurately.

- Look for fasciculation.

- Check the lower spine for scars and the buttocks for wasting.

- Note whether there is pain in the groin, hip or knee (referred pain) region when the patient stands on one leg (allow patients to hold onto your hands for stability), which suggests hip pathology. Confirm by looking for pain on passive rotation of the hip with the patient supine. In severe cases, the hip remains flexed when the patient lies down.

Tone

Test tone in the lower limbs. This will be normal in lesions of the peripheral nerves and muscles and increased in corticospinal lesions.

Power, coordination and reflexes

Test hip flexion and extension, *abduction and adduction*, knee flexion and extension, ankle dorsiflexion and plantar flexion, eversion and inversion. Iliopsoas is tested by asking the patient to flex the hip from a starting position of 90 degrees flexion of the hip (and knees), either when supine or seated. Lifting the leg up from the bed when the patient is supine can be achieved with the use of quadriceps and mask weakness of iliopsoas. Ask the patient to run the heel up and down the shin on each leg in turn. Test the knee, ankle and plantar reflexes.

You are likely to find one of the following patterns of abnormality:

- Weakness of iliopsoas and weakness and wasting of quadriceps. The knee jerk is reduced or absent. Power in the hip adductors is normal (see Box 4.1). The patient has a femoral nerve lesion (Figure 4.1). There may also be sensory impairment over the thigh and medial aspect of the shin. An important cause of a painful femoral nerve lesion is adult-onset diabetes mellitus (diabetic amyotrophy). Haemorrhage into the psoas as a result of anticoagulant therapy and traction during hip surgery are other causes.

---

2. Sir William Gowers, Queen Square neurologist, author of *Diseases of the Nervous System*, the 'Bible' for neurologists for many years (1845–1915).

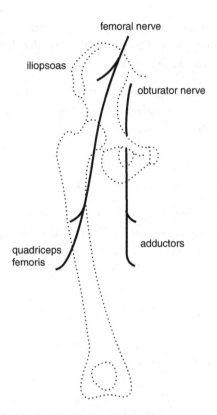

femoral nerve

iliopsoas

obturator nerve

quadriceps
femoris

adductors

Figure 4.1 Muscles supplied by the femoral and obturator nerves.

- Weakness of iliopsoas, quadriceps and hip adductors. The knee jerk is reduced or absent. The patient has an L2/3/4 root or plexus lesion. There is likely to be sensory loss in the equivalent dermatomes. If the lesion involves the cauda equina within the vertebral canal, both legs are likely to be involved. The most likely cause is a tumour, either primary or secondary. Prolapse of an intervertebral disc is uncommon at this spinal level. There are many causes of an upper lumbar plexus lesion, including pelvic malignancy, obstetric injury and neuralgic amyotrophy.

- Weakness of one leg, most marked in hip flexion, knee flexion, ankle dorsiflexion and eversion. Tone and reflexes are increased. The patient has a corticospinal lesion. Perform screening tests on the face and arm looking for evidence of a hemiparesis.

- Weakness of both legs, most marked in hip flexion, knee flexion, ankle dorsiflexion and eversion. Tone and reflexes are increased. The patient has a paraparesis. The lesion is likely to be in the spinal cord. Look for a motor and sensory level.

- Diffuse weakness of the proximal muscles of both legs. Check power and reflexes in the upper limbs. If there is also proximal weakness of the arms, your assessment will largely hinge on the reflex findings:

- Reflexes are preserved or reduced. Consider a myopathy (e.g. muscular dystrophy or polymyositis) or myasthenia gravis (check for fatigability). Inclusion body myositis is one of the most common causes of chronic myopathy in older patients. There is characteristic selective involvement of the quadriceps over other thigh muscles, combined with weakness of the deep finger flexors. The ankle dorsiflexors may also be prominently affected. In Kennedy's disease, there is prominent bulbar weakness (a bulldog face) in addition to proximal lower limb weakness. Look for associated mild sensory neuropathy, chin myokymia, postural tremor and gynecomastia.
- Reflexes are lost. Consider spinal muscular atrophy or myasthenic syndrome (Eaton-Lambert[3] syndrome). The reflexes are also lost in Guillain-Barré syndrome, but here there is likely to be distal as well as proximal weakness.
- Reflexes are increased. Consider MND (check for fasciculation, wasting and fasciculation of the tongue, sensation) or causes of a quadriparesis such as multilacunar state (check gait, jaw jerk, speech, mental state) or cervical myelopathy (normal cranial nerves; loss of some reflexes in the arms, depending on the level).

- Other patterns of proximal weakness are much less common. Weakness confined to hip adduction is seen with obturator nerve lesions (obstetric injury). Selective lesions of the superior gluteal nerve (which supplies gluteus medius and minimus and tensor fasciae latae) and of the inferior gluteal nerve (which supplies gluteus maximus) are very uncommon indeed. Sciatic nerve lesions are a cause of distal weakness of the leg, with or without weakness of hamstrings.

Box 4.1	Tips

- Arthritis of the hip or knee can cause wasting and weakness of quadriceps and diminution or loss of the knee jerk.
- Pain and wasting of quadriceps can be the presenting symptom of adult-onset diabetes mellitus.
- Weakness and wasting of quadriceps can be due to a femoral nerve lesion or an L2/3/4 root (or plexus) lesion. To distinguish between the two, you need to test a muscle which has the same root, but a different nerve supply. The hip adductors fulfil this requirement being supplied by L2/3/4 but via the obturator nerve.

---

3. LM Eaton, American neurologist at the Mayo Clinic (1905–1958).

5 Foot drop

Inspection 26
Tone 28
Power, coordination and reflexes 28

Patients with foot drop often present with falls, as their toes fail to clear the ground.

Foot drop is due to weakness of the tibialis anterior, a muscle supplied by the common peroneal nerve and L4/5 roots. The common peroneal nerve also supplies the peroneal muscles, which evert the foot; the L4/5 roots also supply tibialis posterior, which inverts the foot. Weakness of the tibialis anterior can result from lesions of the corticospinal tract, as well as from lesions of the peripheral nerves or roots.

Inspection

● **Gait**. Get the patient to walk in an open space where the arms can swing freely. The foot is plantar-flexed and inverted and the gait high stepping in a common peroneal nerve lesion. In a corticospinal lesion, the foot is also inverted, but the leg swings in an arc, allowing the toe to clear the ground (circumduction). In a patient with a stroke, the arm may fail to swing. The high stepping gait of foot drop from lower motor neurone pathology occurs because power in the hip flexors is preserved, allowing the patient to appropriately flex the hip more than usual to allow the toe to clear the ground during the swing phase. Foot drop with upper motor neurone pathology is associated with circumduction because reduced knee bend from spasticity and/or weakness of hip flexion prevents effective compensation via exaggerated hip flexion. Ankle flexion dystonia is sometimes confused with foot drop, but the former is associated with active contraction of gastrocnemius and posterior tibialis muscles, whereas the latter is associated with weakness of tibialis anterior. Ask the patient to stand on their toes and then their heels to look for subtle weakness that may not be evident when strength is tested against your own hand. Ask the patient to walk backwards (taking appropriate care): the foot drop may disappear if due to ankle flexion dystonia.

DOI: 10.1201/9781003119166-5

📹 **See Video 10 Common peroneal nerve lesion**
Causing foot drop and high-stepping gait on left.

📹 **See Video 11 Hemiparetic gait following stroke**
Circumduction of the right leg and flexion of the right arm with loss of arm swing.

- **Wasting**. Remove all clothing from the patient's lower limbs after checking that they are wearing an undergarment. Observe the skin, joints and posture, and look for wasting. Wasting is most obvious in the tibialis anterior in a common peroneal nerve lesion. This is seen as a loss of the normal convexity lateral to the ridge of the tibia and is easily missed in a patient lying on a couch if the knees are not lifted. If the calf muscles are also wasted, a number of conditions need to be considered (see the following).

- **Pes cavus** (Figure 5.1). This sign tells you that the lesion is long-standing. Causes include Charcot-Marie-Tooth[1] disease, Friedreich's[2] ataxia and spina bifida.

- **Fasciculation**.

- **The lower spine**. This should be inspected for evidence of spina bifida (lipoma or tuft of hair), spinal deformity or previous surgery.

- Ask the patient to lie on the couch and fully dorsiflex both feet. This is useful for detecting mild unilateral foot drop.

- Check the legs for scars or bruises, particularly over the head of the fibula in a patient with unilateral foot drop.

---

1. Jean-Martin Charcot, French neurologist at the Salpetriere, Paris, one of the founders of the discipline of neurology (1825–1893); Pierre Marie, French neurologist (1853–1940); Howard Henry Tooth, Queen Square neurologist (1856–1926).
2. Nikolaus Friedreich, German pathologist and physician (1825–1882).

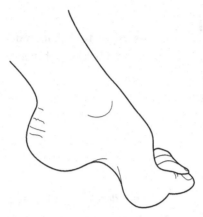

Figure 5.1 Pes cavus.

Tone

Test tone at the knees and look for clonus at the ankles in both legs. Tone is normal in peripheral nerve and root lesions and increased in lesions of the corticospinal tract.

Power, coordination and reflexes

Check hip flexion and extension, knee flexion and extension, ankle dorsiflexion, plantar flexion and inversion and eversion in both legs. Get the patient to run each heel in turn up and down the shin. Test the knee, ankle and plantar reflexes. There are four common patterns of weakness:

- Weakness of dorsiflexion and eversion. The patient has a common peroneal nerve lesion (Figure 5.2), and there will also be weakness of extensor hallucis longus. Reflexes in the leg will be normal, and there may be the typical sensory loss (Figure 5.3). Look for scars or bruising over the head of the fibula. In the rare lesion of the deep peroneal nerve, eversion is normal and the area of sensory loss very small (Figure 5.4).

- Weakness of dorsiflexion, eversion and inversion. The patient has an L4/5 root or plexus lesion. Causes of this include a prolapsed intervertebral disc, tumour of the cauda equina and obstetric injury to the lumbosacral trunk (Figure 5.5). Reflexes in the leg are likely to be normal. There may also be weakness of knee flexion, hip abduction and sensory symptoms or signs in the L4/5 dermatomes (Figure 5.6).

- Weakness of all movements of the foot with normal power at the knee and hip. There are several possibilities:
  - Peripheral neuropathy (with distal weakness of both legs, areflexia and glove and stocking sensory loss).

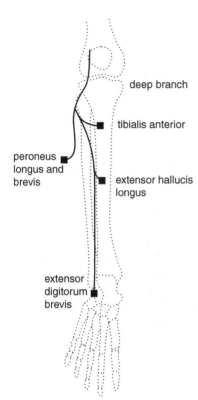

Figure 5.2 Muscles supplied by the common peroneal nerve.

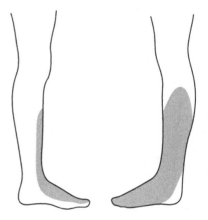

Figure 5.3 Sensory loss in a common peroneal nerve lesion.

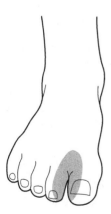

Figure 5.4 Sensory loss in a lesion of the deep branch of the common peroneal nerve.

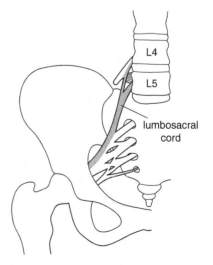

Figure 5.5 The lumbosacral cord arising from the L4, L5 roots.

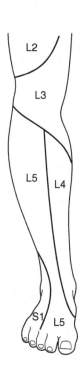

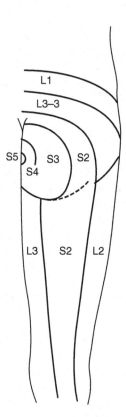

Figure 5.6 Dermatomes of the lower leg.   Figure 5.7 Dermatomes of the buttock.

- Sciatic nerve lesion (rare) due to pressure, trauma, vasculitis or tumour (with loss of the ankle jerk, extensive sensory loss and, depending on the site of the lesion, weakness of the hamstrings).
- Root or plexus lesion (with loss of the ankle jerk and anal reflex, saddle anaesthesia (Figure 5.7) and urinary incontinence). The cauda equina may be involved by tumour or prolapsed disc and the plexus by tumour or trauma.
- Anterior horn cell disease due to MND (with wasting, fasciculation, hyperreflexia and normal sensation).

● Weakness of hip flexion, knee flexion, dorsiflexion and eversion. Tone in the leg is increased and the reflexes are brisk. The patient has a lesion of the corticospinal tract. The following patterns of signs are useful in localizing the site of the lesion:

- Both legs are weak (paraparesis). This is usually due to a spinal cord lesion. If this is in the thoracic cord (e.g. due to a meningioma), the arms will be spared, and there will be a sensory level on the trunk. If it is due to a cervical cord lesion, there will be a loss of reflexes at the appropriate level (C5/6: biceps and brachioradialis; C7/8: triceps), or brisk upper limb reflexes as well with a high cervical cord lesion above C5. Parasagittal tumours pressing on the motor strips of the cerebral hemispheres are a rare cause of weakness in both legs.

- One leg is weak. Possibilities include (1) Brown-Séquard[3] syndrome: check for dissociated sensory loss in the other leg (see Box 5.1) and (2) anterior cerebral artery occlusion: check for a grasp reflex in the hand on the same side. If it is the right leg which is weak, the patient may be aphasic.
- The arm and leg are weak on the same side (hemiparesis). The lesion is likely to be above the cervical cord. The most common causes are a stroke or tumour in the contralateral cerebral hemisphere.

Box 5.1   Tips

- Pes cavus is a useful sign as long as it is not overdiagnosed. It is not enough to have a high arch. There should also be clawing of the toes, and the foot should be thick (see Figure 5.1). These signs are most apparent when the foot is dependent (hanging). If a flat surface is placed against the sole of the foot, a gap is apparent both on the medial and lateral border.

- In testing eversion and inversion of the foot, prevent the patient from rotating the hip by immobilizing the shin with one hand. With the other hand, move the foot into the required position, for example into the fully inverted position, and ask them to hold it there. Then attempt to evert the foot.

- In any patient with absent ankle jerks, it is important to test perineal sensation, as in lesions of the cauda equina sensation elsewhere may be normal.

- Absence of the ankle jerk is a key sign. Take time to put the patient at ease. Use the Jendrassik[4] manoeuvre. Sometimes, the reflex can be obtained more readily by tapping the sole of the foot than by tapping the Achilles tendon. If you are still in doubt, ask the patient to kneel on a chair and tap the tendon while gently dorsiflexing the foot.

- Remember: the spinal cord ends at the second lumbar vertebra. Lesions above this will cause increased tone and reflexes, below it decreased tone and areflexia.

- Selective nerve lesions often occur in the setting of a generalized peripheral neuropathy. In diabetes, for example, a patient may have a foot drop with the typical distribution of weakness of a common peroneal nerve lesion. In addition, the ankle jerk may be lost due to an underlying peripheral neuropathy. Peripheral neuropathy predisposes nerves to pressure palsy.

- A sign of particular importance is dissociated sensory loss where the patient can feel the lightest touch in the affected area but is unable to distinguish one end of a pin from the other. Selective involvement of the pain (spinothalamic) pathways is a feature of syringomyelia, hemi-cord lesions (Brown-Séquard syndrome) and lateral medullary syndrome.

---

3. Charles Edouard Brown-Séquard, Mauritian-born neurologist who practised at Queen Square and later Paris (1817–1894).
4. E Jendrassik, Hungarian neurologist (1858–1921).

- Wasting of extensor digitorum brevis is often found in peripheral neuropathies and in lesions of the common peroneal nerve. In a normal subject, the muscle stands out like a grape when the toes are dorsiflexed against resistance, although wasting is a non-specific finding in the elderly

- Weakness of extension of the great toe may be the only motor sign of an L5 root lesion in a patient with sciatica.

- Spasticity of the legs (increased tone, hyperreflexia, clonus) with well-preserved power (and no sensory loss or bladder involvement) is the characteristic finding in hereditary spastic paraplegia (rare in practice, common in examinations). Hydrocephalus may also cause spasticity of the legs.

6 Ataxia and gait disturbance

Observation 33
Further assessment 34

The observation of gait is probably the single most informative part of the neurological examination. It provides you with an opportunity to see the patient as a whole. Muscle weakness, impairment of balance, sensory loss, involuntary movements, abnormalities of posture, even mood disturbance and dementia may all leave a distinctive imprint on the way we walk. Gait is sadly neglected, yet the extra few moments taken to observe it are rarely wasted. In some diseases, such as Parkinson's disease,[1] the gait is so distinctive that the diagnosis is clear as the patient walks into the room. To benefit from observing gait, you must train your eye to take note of a number of key features (listed in the following section). In this chapter, a number of gaits are described and illustrated on video.

The more you can learn from the gait, the more likely you are to direct the rest of the examination appropriately.

Observation

- Try not to assess gait in a confined space such as a small examination room with a couch in it. You will not be able to judge stride length or arm swing under these conditions. Get the patient to walk in an open corridor. However, if it is not practical to have the patient walk in an open space because of the limitation of space, observing the patient walking back and forth short distances and making a few turns may be sufficient.

- Don't stand too close.

- Don't base your assessment on a couple of strides. Get the patient to walk about 10 metres, turn and come back. In a difficult case, you may want to repeat this.
  - Make particular note of the following:
  - Posture of the head, trunk and limbs

1. James Parkinson, London physician and palaeontologist (1755–1824).

DOI: 10.1201/9781003119166-6

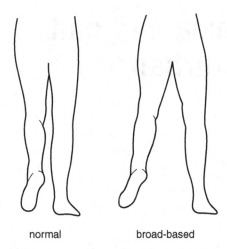

normal   broad-based

Figure 6.1 Normal and broad-based gait (from behind).

- Base or stance (Figure 6.1)
- Stride length
- Step height
- Posture of the leg during the swing phase
- Cadence – the rhythm of the gait, both speed and symmetry
- Arm swing
- Involuntary movements.

● Test tandem gait after unstressed gait, again at least six steps. Tandem gait can be normal even in the very elderly if healthy, but mild instability with advanced age is non-specific.

● Ask the patient to stand on their toes. This is a sensitive test for weakness in gastrocnemius-soleus.

● Ask the patient to stand on their heels. Failure to do this will confirm the presence of foot drop.

● Do the Romberg test (see Box 6.1, page 39).

● If the patient appears to be parkinsonian, check the righting reflex (see the following section).

Further assessment

There are a number of distinctive patterns of gait disturbance:

● One foot is lifted higher than the other during each stride. The affected foot hangs downwards while it is elevated. The patient has a *high-stepping gait* due to unilateral foot drop. This is usually caused by a common peroneal nerve lesion (see section on 'foot drop'). In such a case, the patient will be able to walk on their toes but not on their heel, on the affected side.

See Video 10 Common peroneal nerve lesion
Causing foot drop and high-stepping gait on left.

See Video 12 Spastic gait
Toe-walking spastic gait as a result of hereditary spastic para-paresis in a 21-year-old man.

● Both feet are lifted higher than normal and may produce a slapping sound as they hit the ground. This type of high-stepping gait is most commonly due to bilateral foot drop due, for example, to a peripheral neuropathy such as Charcot-Marie-Tooth disease. MND is another cause. Such patients will have difficulty walking on their toes or heels.

See Video 13 Motor neurone disease
Bilateral high-stepping gait and foot drop due to MND.

● A similar high-stepping gait is seen where there is impairment of sensation in the feet (sensory ataxia). The gait is wide-based and patients watch the ground and their feet intently. Test for Romberg's[2] sign (see Box 6.1, page 39). Place such patients between you and the wall, and ask them to put their feet together and to shut their eyes.

2. Moritz Heinrich Romberg, German physician, author of one of the first textbooks in neurology (1795–1873).

In such a case, the patient may start to fall, without making any apparent attempt to stop themselves. You, of course, must prevent them from falling, but it may be difficult if the patient is very large. You will need to test position sense in the feet. Causes of sensory ataxia include sensory neuropathy, tabes dorsalis, spinocerebellar degeneration and myelopathy, such as from subacute combined degeneration of the cord or multiple sclerosis.

- The shoulders sway from side to side in an exaggerated manner with each stride. The patient appears to be lifting the foot off the ground, not only by flexing the hip and knee but also by tilting the trunk. This is a *waddling gait*. It signifies weakness of hip abduction and can be demonstrated using Trendelenburg's[3] test (Figures 6.2a and b). A positive Trendelenburg sign is defined by a contralateral pelvic drop during a single leg stance. When the left foot is lifted off the ground, the pelvis is normally prevented from tilting downwards on the left side by the action of the right hip abductors. When these are weak, the buttock is seen to sag. It may take a number of

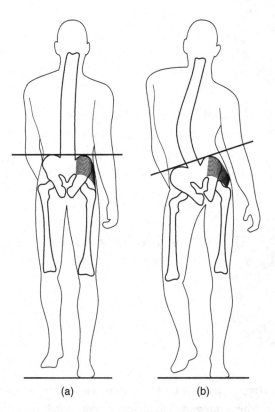

(a)   (b)

Figure 6.2 (a) Normal Trendelenburg test; (b) weakness of right hip abductors.

3. Friedrich Trendelenburg, German surgeon (1844–1924).

seconds before this occurs. Weakness of hip abduction can result from muscle pathology or from disturbance of the normal fulcrum provided by the hip joint. You will need to test proximal muscle power and put the hips through a full range of movements. A waddling gait in a child is likely to be due to muscular dystrophy or congenital dislocation of the hips. In an adult, consider a myopathy and osteoarthritis of the hips.

See Video 14 Antalgic gait and positive Trendelenburg sign in a patient with left sacroiliitis
She minimizes the time that she bears weight on the painful left leg while walking by, hurrying through with the stride on the right. When weight-bearing in the standing position, the pelvis momentarily sags on the right due to failure of the left hip abductors to hold the weight.

- One leg is held stiffly and describes an arc around the other leg with each stride (circumduction). The foot scrapes the ground. The arm on the same side does not swing and is flexed at the elbow. This is a *hemiparetic gait*. There may be obvious facial weakness. You will need to test tone, power and reflexes in the limbs. The most common cause in an adult is stroke.

- Both legs are held stiffly and show circumduction. The steps are short and slow, as though the patient is wading through water. The feet are inverted and may cross ('scissor'). This is a spastic paraparetic or *scissoring gait*. It is seen in its most florid form in long-standing disorders, such as cerebral palsy and hereditary spastic paraplegia. Scissoring is less of a feature when paraparesis is acquired later in life, for example in association with cervical spondylosis or multiple sclerosis.

See Video 11 Hemiparetic gait following stroke
Circumduction of the right leg and flexion of the right arm with loss of arm swing.

See Video 12 Spastic gait

- The patient fails to swing one arm as they walk. The gait is otherwise normal. The patient may have early Parkinson's disease (check for tremor, rigidity and akinesia). Test shoulder joint mobility; a frozen shoulder can also interfere with the arm swing. Patients who have made an otherwise good recovery from stroke may also have reduced arm swing, as can patients with a unilateral antalgic gait from knee or hip pathology.

- The patient is flexed at the neck, elbows, hips and knees. The arms fail to swing. Steps are small and shuffling. Several steps are taken in turning. The base is normal. This is a *parkinsonian gait*. Other features which may be present include hand tremor, which is often exacerbated when a Parkinson's patient walks; increasingly rapid and shorter steps (festination); a tendency to run forwards (propulsion) or backwards (retropulsion); getting suddenly stuck and unable to go on, particularly when changing direction or going through a doorway (freezing). Another form of freezing is start hesitation when a patient with Parkinson's disease has trouble initiating gait after standing up from a chair. Freezing may be overcome with visual and auditory cues and various manoeuvres such as instructing the patients to exaggerate their gait as if they are marching.[4]

See Video 15 Gait in advanced Parkinson's disease
Difficulty getting out of the chair, flexed at the hips, walks slowly with no arm swing; paradoxically, she can still run.

See Video 16 Freezing
Marked freezing in Parkinson's disease overcome by using visual cues.

4. Mirelman A, Bonato P, Camicioli R, et al. Gait impairments in Parkinson's disease. Lancet Neurol. 2019 Jul; 18(7): 697–708.

• Patients with Parkinson's disease often have an impaired righting reflex. This is tested by using the 'pull test': stand behind the patient; warn them that you are going to give their shoulders a tug ('don't let me get you off balance') and then do so. If balance is normal, the patient takes one or two steps back and fully recovers. In mild impairment, the patient usually takes more than two steps back before recovering. In severe cases, the patient runs backwards uncontrollably (i.e. develops retropulsion) or begins to fall. As with Romberg's test, be careful with large patients. You are less likely to end up on the floor with the patient if you stand with your back close to the wall as you do the test.

See Video 17 Pull test with retropulsion in Parkinson's disease
The patient walks well, though with absent arm swing. Runs backwards when pulled from behind.

• The posture is upright, but the arms fail to swing, and the steps are small and shuffling. Several steps are taken in turning. The appearance is similar to Parkinson's disease with one important difference: it is broad-based. Occasionally arm swing can be preserved or even exaggerated. This is called '*marche à petits pas*' (from the French, 'gait with small steps') and is seen particularly in multi-lacunar states (associated with emotional lability, dementia, generalized hyperreflexia, positive jaw-jerk) and normal-pressure hydrocephalus (associated with cognitive impairment and incontinence of urine).

See Video 18 Marche à petit pas due to multiple lacunes (seen on magnetic resonance imaging (MRI))
Small steps, festination (hurrying) when turning and negotiating the doorway. Like parkinsonism, but with a broadened base and shuffling (also referred to as 'magnetic' gait).

See Video 19 Marche à petit pas due to normal-pressure hydrocephalus
Pre-shunt. The patient walks with small steps on a wide base with preserved arm swing and upright posture.

See Video 20 Normal walking
The same patient as in Video 14 walking normally after being shunted.

● The gait is broad-based, with unsteady irregular steps. There is a tendency to veer to one side or the other and to stagger on turning. These are the features of a cerebellar or *ataxic gait*. See if the patient consistently staggers or turns to one side by asking them to march up and down on the spot with their eyes open and then shut. In Unterberger's test, the patient marches on the spot with the arms held out in front with the hands clasped; rotation is observed in a unilateral labyrinthine lesion. Get them to walk heel to toe and to walk around a chair, first one way and then the other. In a lesion of one cerebellar hemisphere, they will consistently stagger to the side of the lesion (look for intention tremor and incoordination in the limbs, nystagmus and dysarthria). In midline cerebellar lesions, the patient will stagger in any direction. The trunk may tilt when the patient is seated. Often, there is no other evidence of cerebellar disturbance, such as intention tremor, nystagmus or dysarthria.

See Video 21 Mild cerebellar ataxia
Broad-based, unsteady on turning, uneven stride.

See Video 22 Progressive dysarthria
Dysarthria, ataxia and limitation of upgaze as a result of SCAIII (Machado–Joseph disease).

● Patients with involuntary movement disorders often have distinctive gaits:

- The patient walks with the head twisted to one side (torticollis).

 See Video 23 Gait in cervical dystonia
The head is tilted to the right as the patient walks.

- The head, trunk and limbs assume bizarre postures, often with associated abnormal movements (e.g. torsion dystonia).

 See Video 24 Gait in torsion dystonia
The patient walks awkwardly and hurriedly with the right arm internally rotated, the left arm flexed at the elbow, the right foot dorsiflexed and the head tilted to the right.

- Constant, random, twitches in all parts of the body interrupt the normal, smooth flow of movement, causing irregular, lurching and staggering. There may be facial grimacing and abnormal posturing of the limbs or trunk. These are features of the gait in Huntington's disease, also often referred to as 'dancing' gait.

 See Video 25 Gait in Huntington's disease
The patient has a curious, untidy, mannered way of walking: bending the knees, pausing and making choreiform movements with his fingers.

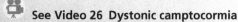

See Video 26 Dystonic camptocormia
Flexion of the trunk with marked improvement following botulinum toxin injections into the rectus abdominus.

See Video 27 Progressive generalized dystonia
Generalized dystonia secondary to DYT1 (TorsinA) mutation.

- There are continuous writhing movements of the limbs during walking; one foot tends to invert, interfering with walking (e.g. 'dopa-induced dyskinesia' in a patient with Parkinson's disease).

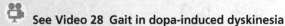

See Video 28 Gait in dopa-induced dyskinesia
As the patient walks, he makes continuous writhing twisting movements of his head, trunk and limbs.

- Patients who experience pain in the leg on bearing weight develop a very characteristic gait. You can see it for yourself by walking in front of a mirror with a pebble in your shoe. Each time you bear weight on the painful side, you hurry through the stride with the good leg to minimize the duration of the pain. The painful leg also buckles each time it bears weight in order to cushion the impact. This is called an *antalgic gait*. It is usually associated with arthritis of the hip, knee, ankle or foot joints.

See Video 14 Antalgic gait and positive Trendelenburg sign in a patient with left sacroiliitis

- A shuffling gait with small steps and loss of arm swing is likely to be due to idiopathic Parkinson's disease if the base is normal. A shuffling gait but with a widened base is seen in vascular parkinsonism and normal-pressure hydrocephalus and the multi-lacunar state. The base is often also widened in the parkinsonian disorder progressive supranuclear palsy (Steele Richardson syndrome).[5] In contrast to the narrow-base, shuffling gait of patients with Parkinson's disease, those with progressive supranuclear palsy tend to pivot on their toes rather than turn en bloc.

- Romberg observed that patients with loss of proprioception due to tabes dorsalis toppled when asked to stand with their feet together and eyes closed. An increase in body sway following closure of the eyes is often accepted as a positive Romberg's sign. Unfortunately, this can occur when balance is impaired for any reason, and even in normal, anxious individuals. The term 'positive Rombergism' is, therefore, better reserved for patients who can stand unassisted but would fall upon closing their eyes if you did not prevent them. Do not attempt this test on a patient who is larger than you are without assistance.

- Most patients who have difficulty in walking will have evidence, when you come to examine them on the couch, of weakness, spasticity, rigidity, akinesia, sensory loss, or ataxia. If none of these is present, consider the possibility of a truncal ataxia due to a midline cerebellar lesion; alcoholism is the most common cause of this. Another possibility is an apraxia of gait due to a frontal lobe lesion.

5. John Steele, Canadian neurologist at Toronto General Hospital then Guam; J Clifford Richardson, Canadian neurologist (1909–1986).

7 Facial weakness

Inspection 45

Distribution of weakness 47

Sensation on the face 49

Taste 50

Other important signs to look for 50

The facial muscles are supplied by the VIIth cranial nerve, which arises from the facial nucleus in the pons (Figure 7.1). The facial nerve is accompanied, for part of its course, by the chorda tympani, which innervates the taste receptors of the anterior two-thirds of the tongue. The muscles of the forehead are represented in the ipsilateral, as well as the contralateral, cerebral hemisphere (Figure 7.2). Stroke is the most common cause of an upper motor neurone facial palsy, and Bell's[1] palsy the most common cause of a lower motor neurone palsy. Other causes of facial palsy are rare. The site of the lesion causing facial palsy is assessed by noting: (1) the pattern of facial weakness and (2) the presence of other signs.

 See Video 29 Bell's palsy

The patient is unable to raise the right eyebrow (frontalis) or screw up the right eye (orbicularis oculi), or smile on the right, or purse his lips on the right (orbicularis oris) or contract the right platysma. When he screws the eyes up, the right eye is seen to roll up (Bell's sign).

 See Video 30 Hemifacial spasm

Right hemifacial spasm in a patient with prior right Bell's palsy showing ipsilateral synkinesis of lower facial muscles when he voluntarily contracts right upper facial muscles.

1. Sir Charles Bell, Scottish anatomist and surgeon (1774–1842).

DOI: 10.1201/9781003119166-7

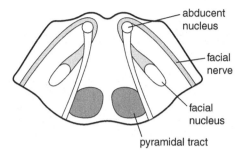

Figure 7.1 Transverse section of the pons.

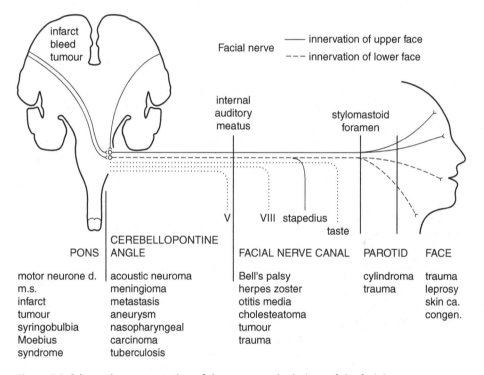

Figure 7.2 Schematic representation of the course and relations of the facial nerve.

Inspection

● Are there vesicles behind the ear, within the external meatus or on the palate (geniculate herpes, the Ramsay Hunt syndrome)?[2]

● Is there evidence of a parotid mass or swelling (cylindroma, sarcoidosis)?

● When the patient blinks, does the corner of the mouth twitch? When the patient smiles, does the eye close more on the affected side? These are features of synkinesis

2. James Ramsay Hunt, American neurologist (1872–1937).

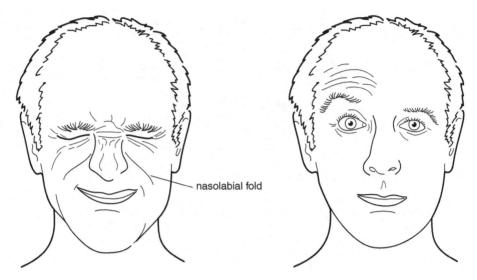
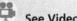
nasolabial fold

Figure 7.3 Raising the eyebrows: selective lesion of the temporal branch of the facial nerve.

('cross-talk' between axons within the facial nerve) and signify that the lesion is long-standing. Pouting is better than smiling for revealing eye closure due to synkinesis.

See Video 31 Long-standing right facial palsy
Deepened right nasolabial fold; spontaneous blinking stronger on the normal (left) side; right corner of the mouth twitches when he blinks; smiling, pouting or blowing his cheeks out all cause the right eye to close; right cheek blows out less than left (tighter right buccinator). All features of overactivity of surviving axons in the right facial nerve associated with synkinesis ('cross-talk' between axons). These signs are not due to contracture of the right facial muscles, as they are lost if the nerve is severed by, for example, surgery for acoustic neuroma.

● Is the nasolabial fold (Figure 7.3) lost (confirming weakness of the facial muscles) or deepened (signifying a long-standing weakness and associated with synkinesis)?

● Look for scars on the face (previous surgery for skin cancers) and over the occiput (previous surgery for acoustic neuroma).

Distribution of weakness

Ask the patient to do the following:

- Raise the eyebrows. Some patients have difficulty doing this voluntarily but will do it involuntarily when asked to look up at the ceiling.

- Screw the eyes up tightly. Observe whether the eyelashes are buried.

- Show you their teeth.

- Blow the cheeks out. Air will escape from the mouth if there is weakness of the orbicularis oris, and the cheek will blow out more on the side where there is weakness of the buccinators.

- Turn the corners of their mouth down. This will also cause platysma to contract in many patients.

There are four main patterns of weakness:

- Weakness of all the muscles on one side of the face except frontalis and orbicularis oculi. The patient has an upper motor neurone lesion. This is most commonly due to a stroke involving the contralateral cerebral hemisphere and the facial weakness is but one part of a hemiparesis (detectable with your screening tests). Patients with this type of facial weakness often elevate the angle of the mouth involuntarily when smiling, but cannot do so on command.

🎥 **See Video 32 Left upper motor neurone facial palsy following stroke**
The patient's face is symmetrical at rest; on being asked to smile, he blinks and closes his eyes (apraxia of smiling) and then fails to elevate the right angle of the mouth fully; later, when amused, he smiles symmetrically.

- Weakness of all the muscles on one side of the face. The patient has a lower motor neurone lesion, usually due to Bell's palsy. In Bell's palsy, there is often loss of taste and hyperacusis but no other signs. If it is due to a lesion of the facial nucleus, the patient may also have a CN VI nerve palsy or gaze palsy on the same side (see Figure 7.2). If it is due to tumour – for example, acoustic neuroma – or infection within the facial nerve canal, there may also be deafness or loss of taste.

- Bilateral facial weakness. When this occurs acutely, it is usually due to Guillain-Barré syndrome, and there may be associated generalized weakness and areflexia. Other causes of bilateral facial weakness or loss of facial movement include:
  - Sarcoidosis (with parotid swelling and fever)

- Myopathies such as facio-scapulo-humeral dystrophy, oculopharyngeal dystrophy or mitochondrial myopathy
- Dystrophia myotonica (with ptosis, wasting of the masseters and sternomastoids, cataracts, frontal balding and inability to release the hand grip)

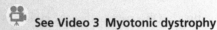 **See Video 3 Myotonic dystrophy**
Frontal balding, ptosis, 'horizontal smile', failure to bury the eyelashes, myotonia causing slowing of fist opening and percussion myotonia of thumb abduction.

- Myasthenia gravis (with ptosis and diplopia which worsen with sustained contraction and rapidly improve with rest. The pupils are spared. There may also be proximal weakness of the limbs).
- Parkinson's disease. The lack of facial expression (hypomimia) in the patient with Parkinson's disease is not due to weakness but to facial akinesia and rigidity. These patients are able to bury their eyelashes and blow their cheeks out. Occasionally facial movements may be asymmetrical because of facial akinesia and/or rigidity on the more affected side, giving rise to apparent weakness. The facial asymmetry will disappear if the patient is given more time to give a full smile.
- Bilateral upper motor neurone facial weakness occurs in multilacunar states (pseudobulbar palsy) and MND. There is usually a brisk jaw jerk. While these patients have difficulty voluntarily contracting the facial muscles, their expressions may change in an exaggerated manner, and they may laugh or cry inappropriately.

● Weakness confined to one or two facial muscles on the same side (rare). In Figure 7.3, for example, weakness is confined to frontalis. This is very rare in acute Bell's palsy; it may occur following incomplete recovery from a Bell's palsy and is then associated with synkinesis. Such a selective weakness is usually due to a lesion of the facial nerve after it has divided into its terminal branches in the parotid gland. Causes include facial trauma, parotid tumour, leprosy and perineural spread from a skin cancer.

 See Video 33 Selective right facial weakness from skin cancer
The right upper lip fails to purse, and the patient is unable to form a seal with his mouth when attempting to blow out his cheeks; he is able to raise his eyebrows and screw up his eyes normally but unable to flare the right nostril. The scar on the right cheek is from previous surgery for squamous cell carcinoma.

Some patients who recover from Bell's palsy develop involuntary movements of the affected side of the face. This post-Bell's hemifacial spasm is usually associated with synkinesis due to aberrant regeneration of the facial nerve.

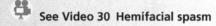

See Video 30 Hemifacial spasm

This form of hemifacial spasm should be differentiated from the more typical hemifacial spasm, usually caused by compression or irritation of the facial nerve by an artery in the posterior fossa.

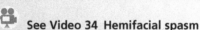

See Video 34 Hemifacial spasm
Right hemifacial spasm and elevation of ipsilateral eyebrow as a result of frontalis contraction, referred to as 'the other Babinski sign'.

Sensation on the face

Test touch and pinprick sensation on the forehead, cheek and chin on both sides of the face. Check corneal sensation. Several types of findings are worth considering:

- It is normal in Bell's palsy. Absence of the corneal reflex in Bell's palsy is due to interruption of the efferent limb of the reflex arc; the other eye blinks briskly when the cornea on the paralyzed side is touched.

- In acoustic neuroma, there is usually loss of corneal sensation, and neither eye blinks when the cornea on the affected side is touched. Facial sensation is otherwise normal. Facial weakness is slight, and there is deafness.

- Facial numbness, as part of a hemianaesthesia, is seen with strokes.

- Loss of sensation on the face, in the distribution of terminal branches of the trigeminal nerve, is a feature of perineural spread from skin cancers.

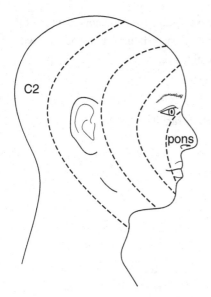

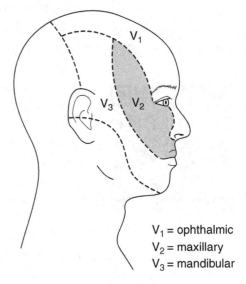

V_1 = ophthalmic
V_2 = maxillary
V_3 = mandibular

Figure 7.4 Onion-peel distribution of sensory loss associated with central lesions of the trigeminal nerve.

Figure 7.5 Distribution of sensory loss associated with peripheral lesions of the trigeminal nerve.

- Loss of sensation in the coolest parts of the face (nose and ears) is characteristic of leprosy (rare).

- Dissociated sensory loss on the face is seen in brainstem lesions, such as syringobulbia or glioma. Pain sensation is lost and touch sensation is preserved. The pattern of sensory loss with central lesions follows an 'onion-peel' pattern (Figure 7.4), unlike sensory loss from peripheral lesions of the trigeminal nerve (Figure 7.5).

Taste

The testing of taste is time-consuming and for this reason often omitted. Taste sensation is normal in upper motor neurone facial weakness and in lesions of the facial nerve after it has left the facial canal. It is often lost in Bell's palsy and other lesions within the facial canal. It should be noted that taste buds (receptors) on the tongue sense bitterness, sweetness, saltiness, sourness and a fifth sensation, 'umami' (savouriness). Complex 'tastes' in food are mediated via olfaction.

Other important signs to look for

- **Ptosis.** The combination of weakness of orbicularis oculi and ptosis, with normal pupillary function, usually signifies that the problem involves muscle or neuromuscular function (see previous discussion).

● **Bilateral ophthalmoplegia**. This again usually signifies muscle disease or myasthenia gravis, with the pupils being spared. Another cause of facial weakness and ophthalmoplegia is the Miller Fisher[3] variant of Guillain-Barré syndrome.

● **Hearing**. The combination of deafness and facial palsy is seen in lesions of the cerebellopontine angle (e.g. acoustic neuroma) or of the facial canal (see Figure 7.2). Hyperacusis often occurs in Bell's palsy due to paralysis of the nerve to stapedius.

● **Facial swelling** (rare) occurs in the Melkersson-Rosenthal[4] syndrome. Here, the facial palsy is often recurrent. Facial swelling also occurs in parotid tumours and parotitis due to sarcoid.

Box 7.1   Tips

● In an acute 'upper motor neurone' facial weakness, frontalis can be weak for a few days and may be difficult to differentiate from 'lower motor neurone' weakness.

● The elevators of the eyelids are not supplied by the facial nerve. Ptosis is not, therefore, a feature of a facial nerve lesion. A confusing sign is narrowing of the palpebral fissure due to overactivity of the orbicularis oculi muscle. This is seen in long-standing Bell's palsy and is associated with deepening of the nasolabial fold and a dimple in the chin, or intermittently during hemifacial spasm.

● Facial palsy, occurring immediately after a fracture of the petrous part of the temporal bone, usually does not improve, as the nerve is severed. When it occurs several days after the head injury, recovery is the rule.

● In multiple sclerosis, facial palsy – unlike weakness in other muscle groups – is often 'lower motor neurone' in type. This may be due to demyelination of the nerve fascicle during its relatively long course within the pons after it forms from the facial nucleus (see Figure 7.1).

● Many patients with Bell's palsy complain of a slight alteration of sensation on the affected side. This can be safely ignored, provided that the patient can feel the lightest touch, tell one end of the pin from the other and has a normal consensual blink reflex.

● The affected eye sometimes brims with tears. This is due to the separation of the punctum of the lacrimal duct from the conjunctival surface. It is not due to excessive production of tears. To the contrary, lacrimation is often reduced in Bell's palsy due to the involvement of parasympathetic nerves.

● Bilateral facial weakness is easy to miss, as the patient's features are symmetrical. It should be suspected when, during the course of giving you the history, the patient is unblinking, expressionless and smiles 'horizontally' – that is, they fail to elevate the angles of the mouth. Speech

---

3. Charles Miller Fisher, Canadian neurologist at the Massachusetts General Hospital (1913–2012).
4. Ernst Gustaf Melkersson, Swedish physician, 1898–1932; Curt Rosenthal, German psychiatrist, twentieth century.

is often impaired – particularly labial sounds like 'puh' – and the patient cannot form a seal with the lips when asked to blow the cheeks out. In severe cases, the eyes are seen to roll up as the patient blinks (Bell's phenomenon).

● Bell's phenomenon is useful for determining whether a patient is really trying to screw the eyes up. Unless there is paralysis of the extraocular muscles, the eyes roll up when the orbicularis oculi muscles contract forcefully.

● Beware the child with an acute Bell's palsy where there is a recognized association with hypertension. Hypertension and diabetes are also risk factors in adult Bell's palsy.

● Finally, do not overdiagnose facial palsy. Many patients have a lopsided smile and they will soon tell you that this has always been the case if you ask them. An old photograph is helpful.

8 Ptosis

Inspection 53
Distribution of weakness 54

Drooping of the eyelids is common in the elderly and results from dehiscence of the levator aponeurosis. Otherwise, it usually results from weakness of the levator palpebrae superioris muscle. This is innervated by the oculomotor (IIIrd) nerve. The under-surface of the levator muscles is connected to the tarsus by smooth muscle fibres, Müller's muscle, which is innervated by cervical sympathetic nerves. Ptosis results from damage to these nerves or to disorders of muscle or neuromuscular junction.

Inspection

Give yourself a moment to take in the overall appearance of the patient. There are some characteristic presentations:

● One eye closed, the other normal (oculomotor palsy or myasthenia gravis).

● Ptosis with lowering of the upper eyelid due to weakness of the levator palpebrae on one side with the pupil larger on the same side (oculomotor palsy; Figure 8.1).

 See Video 35 Third nerve palsy
Trauma-induced left third nerve palsy manifested by ptosis and ophthalmoparesis and contralateral kinetic/postural tremor and ataxia (Benedict's syndrome).

● Partial ptosis with lowering of upper eyelid and elevation of the lower eyelid due to weakness of the Müller's muscle on one side with the pupil smaller on the same side (Horner's syndrome; Figure 8.1).

DOI: 10.1201/9781003119166-8

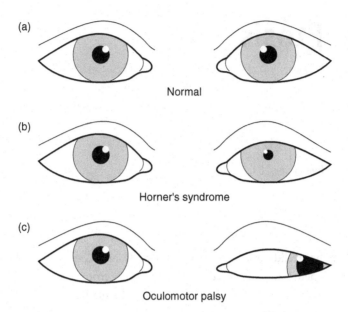

(a)

Normal

(b)

Horner's syndrome

(c)

Oculomotor palsy

Figure 8.1 The eyes in the primary position: (a) normal, (b) Horner's syndrome, (c) oculomotor nerve palsy.

● Bilateral ptosis (myopathy, such as dystrophia myotonica (drooping mouth, thin neck and frontal balding) or mitochondrial disease (e.g. Kearns-Sayre[1] syndrome); or myasthenia gravis).

● Proptosis and ptosis in one eye (orbital tumour or vascular anomaly). Look for dilated conjunctival vessels (carotico-cavernous fistula) and listen for a bruit over the eye.

Distribution of weakness

In the first place, you need to

● test visual acuity;

● test visual fields (ask someone to assist in holding the ptosed eyelid up, or you will erroneously conclude the fields are restricted);

● examine the lens and fundi;

● test pupillary response to light and accommodation;

● test eye movements; and

● examine for weakness of the facial muscles (especially orbicularis oculi). Look for asymmetrical burying of the eyelashes or formation of periocular creases.

1. Thomas P Kearns, Mayo Clinic neuro-ophthalmologist (1922–2011); George Pomeroy Sayre, American ophthalmologist (1911–1992).

What you find will then lead you to other aspects of the examination. Certain patterns of weakness are characteristic:

● **Unilateral ptosis:**
  • With the patient attempting to look straight ahead, the eye is 'down and out' (see Figure 8.1c). There is weakness of adduction and vertical eye movements; the pupil is fixed and dilated. The patient has an oculomotor (IIIrd) nerve palsy (see Chapter 9).
  • As for the previous case, but with pupillary sparing. Consider an ischemic lesion of the oculomotor nerve – e.g. due to diabetes mellitus, hypertension or vasculitis.

📹 **See Video 36 Left oculomotor (IIIrd) nerve palsy with pupillary sparing**
Complete ptosis; the patient is unable to fully adduct left eye on right lateral gaze; then fixates with left eye, causing right eye to abduct (Hering's law); normal abduction with left eye but limited elevation. Pupils equal.

  • With the pupil smaller on the same side but normally reactive to light, eye movements are full (see Figure 8.1b). The patient has a Horner's syndrome. If you look carefully, you may note that the lower lid is elevated on the affected side. Brush the back of your hand across the forehead. The skin may feel moist and sticky on the normal side but smooth on the anhidrotic side. Horner's syndrome is a good lateralizing but a poor localizing sign as the cervical sympathetic fibres run such a tortuous course. The following associated signs should be particularly looked for:
    ● Loss of the corneal reflex in the same eye (orbital or retro-orbital lesion)
    ● Weakness and loss of reflexes in the ipsilateral arm (avulsion injury to the brachial plexus; Pancoast[2] tumour of the lung apex)
    ● Ipsilateral loss of facial pain and temperature sensation and contralateral loss of pain and temperature sensation in the trunk and limbs (brainstem lesion)

  • With (or without) weakness of extraocular muscles and orbicularis oculi consider *myasthenia gravis*. Ask the patient to look up at the ceiling for about 2 minutes. The ptosis may worsen. After a brief rest, the eyelid will resume its original position. Alternatively, ask the patient to forcefully close the eyes for 30 seconds and then open them. In *myasthenia gravis*, the ptosis will be transiently abolished (Bienfang's test), with over 90% sensitivity and specificity. Look for evidence of weakness and fatigability in the limbs. Fatigability is most conveniently tested in the deltoid muscles. Sit the patient in a chair and ask them to abduct the arms at the shoulder,

2. Henry Khunrath Pancoast, American radiologist and radiotherapist (1875–1939).

flex the elbows and to resist your attempts to press their arms down. It is easier for you to sustain this by pressing repetitively (about once per second) rather than continuously. Within a minute or so, it becomes progressively easier to press the arms down if the patient has myasthenia gravis. Again, after a brief rest, the muscle strength returns. Triceps is often weak in myasthenia gravis.

See Video 37 Unilateral ptosis due to myasthenia gravis
Ptosis increases with sustained upward gaze and improves after a brief rest.

● Bilateral ptosis

- With normal pupils. This usually signifies a disorder of muscle or neuromuscular junction. If there is weakness of the extraocular muscles and of the orbicularis oculi, the following should be considered:
  - Senile ptosis (see Box 8.1).
  - Ocular myopathy. In mitochondrial disease such as Kearns–Sayre syndrome, there is complete or partial ophthalmoplegia with ptosis which may be unilateral or asymmetrical, and the pupils are normal. In other myopathies, there may be generalized weakness. Perform an electrocardiograph (ECG) to see if there is a conduction defect.

 See Video 38 Ptosis
Marked left ptosis, bilateral ophthalmoplegia and weakness of orbicularis oculi in Kearns–Sayre syndrome.

  - Myasthenia gravis (see the previous discussion).
  - Dystrophia myotonica. Supporting evidence will include frontal balding, cataracts, wasting of the masseters, sternomastoids and distal limb muscles. Again, check the ECG to see if there is a conduction defect. Test for myotonia (see section on wasting of the hand).

 See Video 39 Ocular myasthenia gravis
Ptosis and divergent squint; on sustained upward gaze, the ptosis increases; later, the ptosis is abolished by injection of edrophonium.

- With unreactive dilated pupils. This uncommon finding is likely to be due to an abnormality of the oculomotor nerves (such as Miller Fisher syndrome) or their central connections in the midbrain. Always ensure the patient has not had eye drops administered for an eye examination!

Box 8.1	Tips

- Complete ptosis, where the pupil is covered by the lid, is unlikely to be due to Horner's syndrome. Furthermore, Horner's syndrome is manifested not only with droopiness of the upper eyelid but also weakness of the lower eyelid as a result of which it is slightly elevated, causing narrowing of the palpebral fissure from below as well as above.

- Pupillary inequality due to an oculomotor palsy is most obvious in a well-lit room; conversely when due to Horner's syndrome, it is most obvious in a dimly lit room.

- Ptosis associated with weakness of orbicularis oculi is likely to be due to myasthenia gravis or to an ocular myopathy.

- Always consider myasthenia gravis when the pattern of weakness of eye movements cannot be readily fitted into a IIIrd, IVth or VIth cranial nerve palsy (and even when it can).

- In unilateral Horner's syndrome which has been present from birth, the iris of the affected eye may remain blue when the other becomes brown (heterochromia).

- In thyroid eye disease, ophthalmoplegia is usually associated with lid retraction, not ptosis.

- A common cause of bilateral ptosis is 'mechanical' ptosis where the levator palpebrae muscle dehisces from the tarsal plate. This condition is seen in elderly patients, and is often called 'senile ptosis'. Look for loss of the fine creases in the upper lid when the patient is attempting to keep the eyes fully open. There are no associated neurological signs.

- In ptosis associated with a complete IIIrd nerve palsy, there is often mild proptosis when the patient is examined sitting up. This is due to loss of tone in the extraocular muscles; it disappears when the patient lies down.

9 Abnormalities of vision or eye movement

Inspection 58
Testing vision 58
The remainder of the examination 63

To see properly, you need to have normal eyes, eye movements and central visual connections. Your approach to the examination thus involves determining which of these three components has failed. The range of possibilities is wide and includes blindness in one eye, bitemporal hemianopia, homonymous hemianopia and IIIrd, IVth or VIth nerve palsies. Patients with pupillary abnormalities and nystagmus will also be considered in this chapter. Many people experience difficulty in testing the eyes, and some time will be spent in describing techniques which are useful.

Inspection

Step back and look at the patient as a whole. Certain features may be very revealing:

- Acromegaly or the smooth, soft, 'feminine' cheeks (in a man) signifying hypopituitarism. In such patients, you will be looking carefully for a bitemporal hemianopia.

- A patient with an obvious hemiparesis may also have a homonymous hemianopia, though this is only one of many associations.

- Loss of facial expression and ptosis raise the possibility of disorders of muscle or the neuromuscular junction (myopathy, myasthenia gravis, dystrophia myotonica).

- Look carefully at the eyes for nystagmus, inequality of the pupils, proptosis, cataracts and evidence of trauma.

Testing vision

Test the following in every patient:

- **Acuity**. Carry a card with letters of different sizes which you give the patient to hold at a comfortable reading distance. See what the patient can read (with reading glasses if they are normally used). Ask them if they wear reading glasses and to use them

DOI: 10.1201/9781003119166-9

if they do. The aim of this part of the exercise is to make sure that the patient is not blind or near-blind in one or both eyes. Subtle abnormalities of visual acuity are not a concern. To save time, ask the patient to read the smallest line they can with one eye, then read the smallest line backwards with the other eye. If they cannot read the chart, check whether they can count fingers, ask whether they can see your facial features or whether they can see only the shape of your head or light/dark.

● **Fundoscopy**. Maximize your chances of seeing something other than the reflection of the light from your ophthalmoscope by dimming the lights in the room, using a narrow beam and using, initially, a low light strength. Get as much practice as you can in using the instrument. The main abnormalities you are looking for include: papilloedema, optic atrophy, cataracts or retinal changes such as diabetic retinopathy, hypertensive retinopathy, haemorrhages and retinitis pigmentosa. If you are unable to visualize the retina, consider the possibility of cataracts or opacities in the cornea or vitreous humour.

● **Fields**. Visual field testing is often done badly and obvious abnormalities missed. The following approach may help:
  • *Peripheral field testing.* Sit in front of the patient, as shown in Figure 9.1. The patient has both eyes open. Hold both of your hands in the upper fields and ask the patient

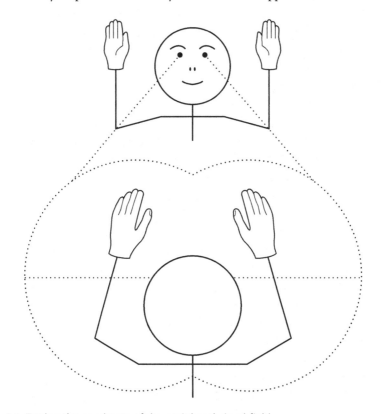

Figure 9.1 Testing the quadrants of the peripheral visual field.

to look at your eyes and to point to where your fingers are moving. Explain that sometimes you will move your fingers on both sides together. Move your fingers on one side, then the other and then both together. Repeat the procedure in the lower fields. This technique is good for detecting homonymous hemianopia and visual inattention or neglect. In the latter, the patient will miss the movements in the affected visual field only when there are simultaneous movements. It is not good at detecting a blind eye, for the field of a single eye is wide.

- *Central field testing* (Figure 9.2). Cup your hand over your left eye and ask the patient to do the same with their right eye (warn the patient not to press on the eye, or it will be untestable for the next few minutes). Ask the patient to look at your eye. Place a red pinhead in each of the four quadrants of the visual field, close to its centre. Ask the patient whether they can see the pin and whether the colour is the same in each quadrant. Don't stray far from the centre of the field; you will see yourself that the colour fades the further out you go. This is a sensitive test for optic nerve and chiasmal lesions; the patient will not see the pin on the affected side, or it will look grey. You can also assess the size of the blind spot in someone with papilloedema.

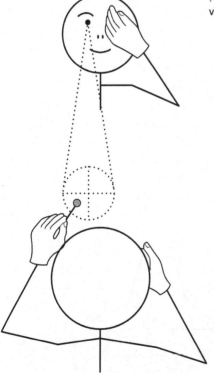

Figure 9.2 **Testing the quadrants of the central visual field with a red pin**

- **Pupillary responses**. See if the pupils are equal. Ask the patient to fixate on the wall opposite and test the direct and consensual light reflexes. An absent light reflex is a key sign and should be checked carefully. A common cause of failure to induce a light reflex on the wards is a flat torch battery. Sometimes it is difficult to see the response in a brightly lit room because the pupils are so constricted. If in doubt, dim the lights. Use the swinging torch test to detect a relative afferent pupillary defect (the Marcus Gunn[1] response): shine the light in one eye and then quickly flick it across to the other eye, wait a second or two and then flick it back. Each time the light hits the eye with impaired vision, the pupil dilates. Test the near reflex.

- **Eye movements**. Observe the position of the eyes and look for evidence of strabismus (squint) or nystagmus in the primary position (looking straight ahead).

  Here are some techniques which may prove useful:

- **Testing eye movements**
  - *Primary gaze position*. Before testing eye movements, it is important to determine whether the patient has a normal primary gaze position. Ask them to look straight ahead. Are the eyes in the midline position or deviated? If deviated, are the eyes conjugate (aligned in the same direction) or disconjugate? Conjugate gaze disorders are supranuclear (but can still arise from lesions in the brainstem – e.g. pons). If disconjugate, is the deviated eye in a position typical for CN III (down and out)? When observing eye movements (see the following), does the misalignment between each eye remain relatively fixed, suggesting a supranuclear gaze palsy, or varies according to the direction of movement, suggesting an internuclear or nerve palsy?
  - There are two major classes of eye movements, saccadic eye movements that voluntarily shift foveal gaze to a target of interest, and pursuit eye movements, which allow you to keep your foveal gaze fixed to a moving target.
  - *Saccadic gaze testing*. First, ask the patient to look to the left, then to the right, then up and then down. This will give you an idea of the range of eye movements and whether they are conjugate or disconjugate, and to form a hypothesis about the nature of the eye movement disorder. Note whether the patient blinks to initiate gaze or moves their head rather than their eyes. With practice, you may notice whether the saccades are slow. (Normal saccades are so rapid you can only see their start and finish.) These disorders of voluntary gaze are characteristic of certain diseases such as progressive supranuclear gaze palsy (PSP), Huntington's disease[2] and the rare spinocerebellar ataxias (SCA II, III and VII). Now, hold the thumb of your left hand and the index finger of your right hand about 50 cm apart in front

1. Robert Marcus Gunn, Scottish ophthalmologist (1850–1909).
2. George Sumner Huntington, American neurologist (1851–1916).

of the patient. Ask the patient to look at your thumb when it moves and then your finger (again, when it moves). See if their eyes can go from one digit to the other in one clean sweep (saccade). The hallmark of motor dysfunction in Parkinson's disease is loss of amplitude of voluntary movements. In the eyes, this is reflected as hypometric saccades, with the eyes moving from thumb to finger in a series of bunny-hops rather than in one leap. In cerebellar disorders, the eyes may overshoot the target and then return (ocular dysmetria). In PSP, the patient may not be able to look down voluntarily and yet will achieve a full vertical excursion if the examiner passively flexes and extends the head as the patient fixates on a target (Doll's eye movement or oculocephalic manoeuvre induced by the vestibulo-ocular reflex).

- *Pursuit gaze testing.* Ask the patient to follow your finger as you trace a large figure 'H'; this causes the eyes to move horizontally and then vertically in the abducted and adducted positions. Check the range of movement achieved by each eye and whether the movements are smooth as they follow your finger; in cerebellar disorders, they are often jerky.

See Video 40 Early PSP (Steele Richardson syndrome)
The patient's range of voluntary eye movements is good, but his vertical saccades, particularly when looking down, are slow.

- **The cover test:**
  - *Objective confirmation of diplopia.* Failure of one or both eyes to move in a certain direction may be obvious. Often it is not, although the patient may complain of seeing double. You may confirm that the eyes are not aligned using the cover test. Ask the patient to fixate on your pin with both eyes open. Move the pin around until you find the position where the patient says that they are seeing double. Now cover each eye in turn. The eye that is fixating will not move when the other is covered. The other eye will move when the fixating eye is covered.
  - The traditional method of determining which muscle is weak is to cover each eye in turn and to ask the patient which of the two images has disappeared. The outer image comes from the eye which has not moved fully. Unfortunately, patients often have difficulty with this test and report that it is the outer image which has gone when either eye is covered. It is more useful to determine from the patient whether the two images are separated in the vertical (e.g. IIIrd and IVth nerve palsies) or horizontal (e.g. VIth nerve palsy) planes.

The remainder of the examination

You now have enough information to proceed with the remainder of the examination. What you do next will depend upon what you have found:

● **Abnormality of vision**. Here, you have found impairment of the visual fields or acuity. This might consist of:
  - **Impairment of acuity in one eye** (Figure 9.3a). Cover the other eye and see if the patient can perceive hand movements or the light of your torch. The pupils are equal, but the affected eye has no response to light or has a relative afferent pupillary defect. The problem lies in the anterior visual system: the eye itself (e.g. central retinal artery occlusion, retinitis pigmentosa) or the optic nerve. If there is swelling of the optic disc, consider conditions such as optic neuritis or acute anterior ischaemic optic neuropathy (feel the superficial temporal pulses and check the erythrocyte sedimentation rate (ESR) as temporal arteritis can cause this; also see Box 9.1, p. 65). If there is optic atrophy, a number of possibilities exist: subfrontal meningioma (test smell), pituitary tumour, carotid aneurysm, past ischaemic optic neuropathy, multiple sclerosis, trauma, syphilis.
  - **Bitemporal hemianopia** (Figure 9.3b). This signifies a lesion of the optic chiasm, most commonly due to a pituitary tumour. You may have already observed the changes of hypopituitarism or acromegaly. Ask the patient if he/she has galactorrhoea (prolactinoma).
  - **Homonymous hemianopia** (Figure 9.3c and f). This signifies a lesion behind the optic chiasm – that is, involving the optic tract, radiation or visual cortex. In a left homonymous hemianopia, look for evidence of non-dominant parietal lobe function. Get the patient to draw a clock, put a cross in the middle of a line and copy a cube. Test for sensory neglect. Use your screening tests to detect a hemiparesis. In a right homonymous hemianopia, look for evidence of aphasia and again for

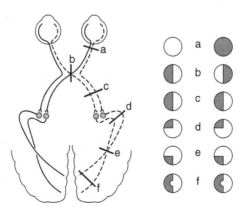

Figure 9.3 **Examples of visual field losses and their associated lesions.**

hemiparesis. Test reading. The most common causes of homonymous hemianopia with these signs are stroke and tumour.

- **Upper homonymous quadrantanopia** (see Figure 9.3d). This signifies a temporal lobe lesion; a **lower homonymous quadrantanopia** signifies a parietal lobe lesion (Figure 9.3e).

- **Abnormality of eye movements**. This is likely to be one of two types:
  - **Weak eye muscles**. Here, there is weakness of the ocular muscles of one or both eyes:
    - The patient fails to abduct one eye (Figure 9.4). There are no other ocular findings. The patient has weakness of the lateral rectus muscle, most commonly due to an abducens (VIth) nerve palsy. The abducens nucleus is in the pons: check facial sensation and use the screening tests, looking for a contralateral hemiparesis (see Figure 7.1). Causes of abducens palsy include microvascular occlusion of the vasa nervorum of the VIth nerve due to hypertension or diabetes, raised intracranial pressure, cavernous sinus lesions and nasopharyngeal carcinoma. Often, no cause is found. Lesions of the abducens nucleus within the

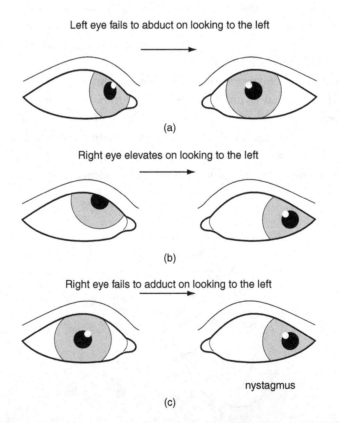

Left eye fails to abduct on looking to the left

(a)

Right eye elevates on looking to the left

(b)

Right eye fails to adduct on looking to the left

nystagmus

(c)

Figure 9.4 (a) Left abducens nerve palsy; (b) right trochlear nerve palsy; (c) right INO.

pons itself do not cause isolated unilateral lateral rectus weakness, but instead, a horizontal conjugate gaze palsy, as the nucleus, is collocated with the pontine centre for lateral gaze.

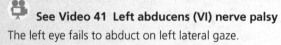

See Video 41 Left abducens (VI) nerve palsy
The left eye fails to abduct on left lateral gaze.

- In the primary position, one eye assumes an abducted and depressed position (see Figure 8.1c). There is weakness of adduction, elevation and depression of the eye and ptosis. The pupil is fixed and dilated. The patient has an oculomotor (IIIrd) nerve palsy. When this occurs acutely and there is eye pain, it is a matter of some urgency to exclude a posterior communicating aneurysm (with a computed tomography (CT) angiogram, magnetic resonance angiogram (MRA) or spiral angiogram). Clipping the aneurysm before it has ruptured carries a much lower mortality than after. Chronic meningitis (e.g. tuberculosis), raised intracranial pressure or cavernous sinus lesions (check trigeminal nerve function) may also cause IIIrd nerve palsies. The pupil is characteristically spared in a IIIrd nerve palsy associated with diabetes mellitus or hypertension.

See Video 36 Left oculomotor (IIIrd) nerve palsy with pupillary sparing
Complete ptosis; the patient is unable to fully adduct left eye on right lateral gaze; then fixates with left eye, causing right eye to abduct (Hering's law); normal abduction with left eye but limited elevation. Pupils equal.

- On looking to the left, the right eye rides up (Figure 9.4b). The head is tilted to the left. The patient has weakness of the right superior oblique muscle, usually due to a trochlear (IVth) nerve palsy. Attempts to demonstrate failure of the eye to depress in the adducted position are usually unrewarding as the IIIrd nerve innervated inferior rectus can still perform this action; however, in an IVth nerve palsy, the eye will fail to intort (rotate). Often, it follows head injury, but diabetes is another cause.

See Video 42 Right trochlear (IV) nerve palsy
The head is tilted to the left; on left lateral gaze, the right eye rides up – this is more marked when the head is tilted to the right and corrected by tilting the head to the left.

- On lateral gaze, one eye fails to adduct (or adducts slowly) and the abducting eye overshoots and then corrects (Figure 9.4c) or shows nystagmus. The affected eye may adduct fully on convergence testing. The patient has a unilateral INO. This signifies a lesion of the medial longitudinal fasciculus (Figure 9.5). Unilateral INO in an older patient is often due to stroke, and bilateral INO usually due to multiple sclerosis.

See Video 43 Left internuclear ophthalmoplegia
On right lateral gaze, the left eye fails to fully adduct, and the right eye overshoots and then makes correcting nystagmoid movements.

- Mild limitation of upward gaze is a common finding in otherwise normal elderly patients and in Parkinson's disease.
- Both eyes fail to look to one side (conjugate gaze palsy). Loss of voluntary lateral gaze usually signifies a lesion of the contralateral frontal lobe or the ipsilateral pons: 'the cortex kicks and the pons pulls' (see Figure 9.5).

See Video 44 Facial and gaze palsy due to pontine metastasis
Widened left palpebral fissure; not blinking on left; loss of left nasolabial fold; unable to raise left eyebrow (frontalis); unable to screw up left eye (orbicularis oculi); left cheek blows out (buccinator weakness); able to look to the right but not the left (left gaze palsy). CT: multiple lesions, including one in the left pons.

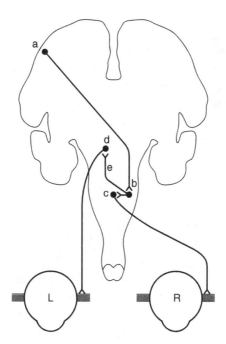

Figure 9.5 Pathway for lateral gaze. (a) Frontal lobe eye field; (b) pontine lateral gaze centre; (c) abducens nucleus; (d) medial rectus nucleus of the oculomotor nerve; (e) medial longitudinal fasciculus.

- On attempted upward gaze, the eyes develop a rapid flickering motion towards each other and retract rhythmically. This is convergence-retraction nystagmus and is a feature of Parinaud's syndrome.[3] The pupils may also become unreactive to light but not to accommodation. The usual underlying cause is compression of the midbrain by a pinealoma. Other causes include hydrocephalus and stroke.

 **See Video 45 Parinaud's syndrome**

On attempted upward gaze, the eyes jerk rhythmically towards each other.

---

3. Henri Parinaud, French neuro-ophthalmologist (1844–1905).

See Video 46 Parinaud's syndrome

On attempted upward gaze, the eyes retract rhythmically into the orbits.

- Loss of downward gaze. In an elderly patient, this is likely to be due to PSP (Steele Richardson syndrome), a type of parkinsonism. Often there is also loss of upward gaze. While the patient cannot look up or down voluntarily or with pursuit, reflex movement is preserved, showing that the lesion is above the nucleus of the oculomotor and trochlear nerves (i.e. it is 'supranuclear'). Ask the patient to look at a point on the wall opposite. Now, tilt the head back (this may be difficult as there is often marked neck rigidity in PSP, in itself a helpful sign) and also forward. This optokinetic manoeuvre can demonstrate full vertical ocular movement indicating that the vertical (downward more than upward) palsy is supranuclear. However, in advanced stages of PSP, this manoeuvre may not overcome the vertical palsy indicating a 'nuclear' component. In patients with early PSP, the supranuclear palsy may not be evident but downward saccades may be impaired as demonstrated by moving the optokinetic nystagmus (OKN) tape or rotating OKN cylinder upward. Another characteristic feature of PSP is square wave jerks, best observed by asking the patient to look at a distant object.

See Video 40 Early PSP (Steele Richardson syndrome)

- **Nystagmus**. This refers to involuntary rhythmical movements of the eyes. In most cases, each movement has a fast and a slow phase ('jerk' nystagmus). Note whether the nystagmus is present in the primary position (looking straight ahead), on horizontal gaze or on vertical gaze. Does it beat in a horizontal (left or right) or vertical plane (up or down)? By convention, the direction of nystagmus is defined by the direction of the fast phase. Vestibular nystagmus can be either 'peripheral' (labyrinth) or 'central' (vestibular nucleus/cerebellum) and is often induced by head movement. Peripheral nystagmus almost always has a torsional (rotatory) component, and central nystagmus (unless due to vestibular nucleus pathology) usually is purely horizontal and/or vertical. Patients with peripheral nystagmus may have deafness and tinnitus, but usually no other signs. Gaze-evoked nystagmus is typically due to brainstem or cerebellar lesions. Several examples of nystagmus are worthy of mention.

- A few beats of horizontal nystagmus, only present at the extremes of lateral gaze. Unsustained nystagmus of this type is physiological. Avoid moving the eyes beyond the range of comfortable binocular vision.

See Video 47 Horizontal nystagmus

On left lateral gaze, there is horizontal nystagmus with the fast phase to the left; on right lateral gaze, there is horizontal nystagmus with the fast phase to the right.

- Fine horizontal nystagmus with the fast component to one or other side, only present on deviation of the eyes to that side. This could be due to a peripheral or central lesion. Peripheral vestibular nystagmus beats away from the side of the lesion, whatever the direction of the gaze. Cerebellar nystagmus is gaze-evoked and typically beats to the side of the lesion if unilateral, but may also beat in whichever direction the patient looks. Central vestibular nystagmus, if purely horizontal, will usually beat away from the side of the lesion whichever way the patient looks. In such a patient you should do the following:
  - Test hearing. Whisper a number on one side while masking the other ear by rubbing the tragus against the external meatus. Hearing might be impaired in a peripheral lesion as in Meniere's[4] disease. It might also be impaired in a cerebellopontine angle tumour. If hearing is impaired, you should do Rinné[5] and Weber[6] tests though, in the noisy environment of a ward or clinic, these are rarely helpful.
  - Test facial and corneal sensation and look for facial weakness (cerebellopontine angle tumour or pontine lesion).

4. Prosper Meniere, French otologist (1799–1862).
5. Heinrich Adolf Rinné, German otolaryngologist (1819–1868).
6. Ernst Heinrich Weber, German anatomist and physiologist (1795–1878).
7. Karl Wernicke, German neuropsychiatrist (1848–1905).

- — Look for cerebellar signs: dysarthria, intention tremor, ataxic gait.
- — Perform screening tests for a hemiparesis.
- Sustained horizontal nystagmus on lateral gaze in both directions. This is seen in patients who are intoxicated with drugs, such as phenytoin, benzodiazepines and barbiturates. They may also have dysarthria and limb ataxia. It may also result from the lesions of the cerebellum and brainstem mentioned.
- Vertical nystagmus. This usually signifies a central lesion. It can be caused by the same drugs as horizontal nystagmus. There are two main types of vertical nystagmus:
  - — Upbeat nystagmus, where the fast phase is upwards. Causes include multiple sclerosis, stroke, tumour and Wernicke's[7] encephalopathy. It is also seen in bilateral INO.
  - — Downbeat nystagmus, where the fast phase is downwards, is less common and is particularly associated with lesions of the cervicomedullary junction, such as the Arnold-Chiari[8] malformation.

See Video 48 Vertical nystagmus
Vertical nystagmus on downward gaze, fast phase down.

- — Nystagmus confined to one eye ('ataxic' nystagmus) is seen in an INO (see above).

See Video 43 Left INO

---

8. Julius Arnold, German physician (1835–1915); Hans Chiari, Austrian pathologist (1851–1916).

- Convergence-retraction nystagmus is seen in lesions of the tectal plate of the midbrain (see the previous discussion).

 **See Video 45 Parinaud's syndrome**

- In pendular nystagmus, there are no clearly recognizable fast and slow phases; the movements are sinusoidal. It is often long-standing and associated with failure of visual fixation or blindness. A common cause is multiple sclerosis.

 **See Video 49 Horizontal pendular nystagmus**
This is present continuously in the primary position and increases in amplitude on lateral gaze. No fast and slow phase.

● **Pupillary abnormality**. This is likely to be one of the following:

- One pupil is smaller than the other. Both react briskly to light and accommodation. There is ptosis on the side of the small pupil. The patient has Horner's syndrome (see Figure 8.1b).
- One pupil is larger than the other. The larger pupil is unreactive to light or accommodation. There is ptosis and limitation of eye movements on the side with the larger pupil. The patient has a IIIrd nerve palsy (see Figure 8.1c).
- One or both pupils are mid-size, react poorly to light, but do constrict to a near stimulus. There is no ptosis; eye movements are full. This is likely to be an Adie[9] ('tonic') pupil; check for areflexia. If more widely dilated, other possibilities include traumatic iridoplegia and the result of a previous application of mydriatic eye drops.
- Both pupils are small, irregular and unreactive to light. The response to accommodation is preserved. There is no ptosis. Eye movements are full. The

9. William John Adie, Queen Square neurologist (1887–1935).

patient may have Argyll Robertson[10] (A-R) pupils. A-R pupils are now rare and more likely due to diabetic autonomic neuropathy than neurosyphilis; more common is a long-standing Adie pupil which eventually becomes small. Like the A-R pupil, the response to accommodation is often brisk and, while the pupil does constrict to light, this may take so long as to be missed. The pupils of patients with glaucoma treated with pilocarpine eye drops are very small, and in these, it may be difficult to see any response to light or accommodation.

Box 9.1   Tips

- Optic nerve disease does not cause inequality of the pupils, for the direct and consensual light reflexes are of equal strength. Thus, if the right optic nerve were transected, the size of the right pupil would remain the same as that of the left, by the action of the consensual reflex.

- The finding of an afferent pupillary defect usually indicates a lesion of the optic nerve and is less common in retinal lesions.

- Optic disc swelling may be due to optic neuritis, raised intracranial pressure or acute anterior ischemic optic neuropathy. In optic neuritis, there is a central scotoma, impairment of colour vision (especially to red) and visual acuity is impaired; in raised intracranial pressure, the blind spots are enlarged and the visual acuity is usually normal in the early stages.

- Myasthenia gravis may mimic a IIIrd, IVth or VIth cranial nerve palsy, and even an INO. The pupil is spared, and there is often weakness of the orbicularis oculi. The signs are usually bilateral and there is ptosis. Fatigability is the key sign.

- Dysthyroid eye disease should always be considered if the abnormality of eye movement does not readily conform to a IIIrd, IVth or VIth cranial nerve palsy. Associated features include proptosis, lid lag, lid retraction and conjunctival injection.

- You will miss the important sign of visual neglect, usually signifying a non-dominant parietal lesion, unless you routinely test the patient with simultaneous stimuli in each half field.

- The obliques elevate and depress the eyes in the adducted position, the recti in the abducted position.

- Abnormalities of conjugate horizontal gaze are seen in lesions of the pons, frontal or occipital lobes. Conjugate vertical gaze is impaired in lesions of the midbrain.

- Nystagmus is likely to be of central origin if it is vertical or involves only one eye.

- Nystagmus, dysarthria and tremor are some of the acute effects of alcohol. Often the only cerebellar sign in a chronic alcoholic is unsteadiness of gait.

- In a young woman, who looks well and has no ocular signs apart from a dilated, slowly reactive pupil, consider Holmes-Adie syndrome.[11] Often, the pupil is oval. Both pupils may be involved. Check the tendon reflexes. In elderly patients with this syndrome, the pupils may become small.

---

10. DMCL Argyll Robertson, Scottish ophthalmologist (1837–1909).
11. Sir Gordon Holmes, Queen Square neurologist whose system of neurological examination forms the basis of what we all do to this day (1876–1965).

In addition to convergence insufficiency, noted with a variety of neurodegenerative disorders, including Parkinson's disease and aging, patients should be tested for convergence spasm, manifested by transient dysconjugate gaze with asymmetric ocular convergence, miosis and accommodation evoked by examination of horizontal gaze mimicking abducens palsy. The latter is particularly common in patients with functional movement disorders.[12]

12. Waln O, Jankovic J. Neuro-ophthalmology of movement disorders. Expert Review of Ophthalmology 2018;13(5):283–292.

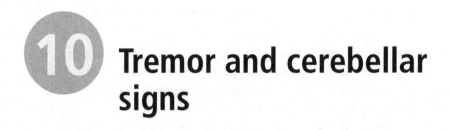

10 Tremor and cerebellar signs

Inspection 74
Examination of tremor 75
Other aspects 77

Tremor is an involuntary, rhythmical, oscillatory movement of any part of the body, but most commonly of the hands. It is convenient to divide tremors into three main categories: resting, postural and intention. The most common cause is physiological tremor, which we all have at times. The patient whose tremor is severe enough to seek medical attention is most likely to have essential tremor, Parkinson's disease, a dystonic tremor syndrome or cerebellar disease.

Inspection

Step back and look at the patient as a whole. You should have two questions in your mind:

● Which parts of the body are shaking? Look particularly at the lips, tongue, chin, head and limbs. Also, ask the patient to make the 'ahhh' sound to listen for any voice tremor, which typically presents in patients with essential tremor. All patients with a history of tremor should be asked to write or perform other activities that typically trigger the tremor. Some patients with task-specific tremor shake only when writing (primary writing tremor), applying make-up, putting while playing golf, texting or performing other activities that require fine coordinated movement.

 See Video 50 Primary writing tremor
Task-specific or task-exacerbated variant of essential tremor without postural tremor in an elderly woman with a 30-year history of handwriting tremor in the right hand that later spread to the left hand, with mild head tremor.

DOI: 10.1201/9781003119166-10

- Are there any signs of parkinsonism, such as rest tremor, hypomimia, bradykinesia, rigidity, decrementing amplitude on rapid succession movements, decreased arm swing, stooped posture and other parkinsonian signs?

Examination of tremor

The next step is to define the characteristics of the tremor. This is done on the basis of the observation of the tremor at rest, while the arms are outstretched in front of the body and in a wing-beating position, and in the finger-to-nose manoeuvre. Patients with essential tremor typically have hand action tremor (during movement) and postural tremor that is evident immediately after assuming an anti-gravity, horizontal, posture. In contrast, patients with Parkinson's disease typically have tremor at rest which, following a latency of several seconds or even as long as a minute, may recur after assuming a horizontal position, the so-called re-emergent tremor.

- The circumstances in which it is maximal.

- Whether it is coarse (high amplitude, low frequency) or fine (low amplitude, high frequency).

Observe the tremor in the hands:

- With the patient sitting with their hands resting on their lap. A tremor that is maximal in this posture is called a **resting tremor** and is characteristic of Parkinson's disease. It is usually coarse and more marked in one hand than in the other. It pauses during movement of the affected hand yet, characteristically, persists or even increases during walking.

See Video 51 Resting tremor in Parkinson's disease
Hand tremor persisting during walking in a patient with Parkinson's disease.

See Video 52 Resting tremor in Parkinson's disease
A highly coordinated synchronous rhythmical contraction in the plane of flexion and extension is seen in the fingers of the left hand. In the right hand, the tremor is pill-rolling, the thumb rubbing against the index. A side-to-side tremor of similar frequency is seen in the jaw.

● With the arms outstretched in front, first with the elbows extended and then flexed with the fingers held in front of the nose. A tremor in this position is called a **postural tremor**. This may be of two types:

- Physiological tremor: a fine tremor present equally in the two hands. It is enhanced by anxiety, after exercise, thyrotoxicosis and adrenergic drugs.
- Essential tremor: this is also usually fine and symmetrical but can be coarse, especially in older patients. It persists during movement.

 See Video 53 Postural tremor in essential tremor
Fine tremor of the outstretched arms; this goes when the arms are at rest and persists during movement; no akinesia of the hands.

● As the patient repeatedly touches their nose and then your finger with each hand in turn. This manoeuvre elicits an **intention tremor**, the development or worsening of tremor as the hand approaches its target. When coarse and appearing only with intention, this often signifies cerebellar dysfunction.

 See Video 50 Primary writing tremor

 See Video 54 Parkinson's disease
Parkinson's disease and childhood-onset hereditary chin tremor.

See Video 55 Intention tremor
A coarse (high-amplitude, low-frequency) tremor is seen in the right hand as the index finger approaches the pointer and the patient's nose.

See Video 56 Intention tremor in cerebellar disease
The patient develops a coarse tremor of the hand as her finger approaches her nose, especially on the right side; there is clumsiness (ataxia) of the hands when she slaps her thighs.

Other aspects

What you do next will be determined by what you have found:

● **Resting tremor**. Your aim is to examine for any additional parkinsonian features u:
  • *Tone*. Test tone in the arms (see Introduction). In Parkinson's disease, tone is increased throughout the range of movement. The tremor may also be felt as 'cogwheeling'.
  • *Akinesia*. This is tested by getting the patient to
    • tap the tips of the extended thumb and index finger repetitively looking for slowing, decrement (progressive loss of amplitude) or motor blocks (interruptions to or sudden reduction in the amplotide of the repetitive movements); and
    • open and close the hand repeatedly with the fingers extended. The amplitude of the movement decreases as the test continues.

See Video 57 Tremor, akinesia and gait in Parkinson's disease
While sitting, there is a coarse tremor of the right hand, causing flexion and extension at the wrist. The tremor pauses briefly when he raises the arms. There is slowing of voluntary flexion and extension of the hands (bradykinesia). The chin shakes. He does not swing the (tremulous) right arm on walking.

- If these tests are performed only with difficulty, make sure that the problem is not due to weakness. Rapid finger movements are also impaired in patients with hemiparesis but do not show the progressive decrement in amplitude which characterizes this activity in Parkinson's disease. Muscle strength is normal in Parkinson's disease.
- *Gait.* Check for loss of arm swing, stooped posture, small steppage and stiffness or hesitation on turning. Eventually, there is loss of balance (demonstrated by performing the 'pull test') and freezing resulting in falls.

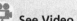 **See Video 58 Falls in Parkinson's disease**
The patient walks cautiously with small steps and with a coarse tremor of the right hand. When he crosses the shadow thrown by light coming through the doorway, he freezes and falls to his knees.

- *Speech.* This will typically be of low volume with a tendency for words to run into each other or to stutter (palilalia).

 See Video 59 Speech in Parkinson's disease
A quiet voice with a tendency to stutter (palilalia).

- **Postural tremor** (essential tremor or enhanced physiological tremor). The first task here is to exclude Parkinson's disease, which is not always easy as in some patients with severe, coarse essential tremor, the tremor persists at rest, especially if the limb is not truly at rest. Conversely, postural tremor is common in Parkinson's disease. Distribution of the tremor, however, is often useful in differentiating the two disorders. Thus, head, voice and handwriting tremor are typically present in patients with essential tremor but not in patients with early Parkinson's disease. On the other hand, patients with Parkinson's disease, in addition to typical rest hand tremor, may also have leg and chin tremor. Another useful way of distinguishing between the two conditions is by observing the gait. In essential tremor, the gait is normal, although some patients may have difficulties with tandem gait. In contrast, in Parkinson's disease (unless in the very early stages or when they are receiving treatment), the gait is almost always abnormal. Furthermore, in essential tremor, the face is expressive, and the patient gesticulates fluently in conversation, the tremor is long-standing, improves with alcohol and there is usually a positive family history of tremor (or alcoholism).

- If it is of recent onset, check for evidence of thyrotoxicosis: tachycardia, sweating, lid lag, exophthalmos, goitre, thyroid bruit, weight loss. Enquire about what drugs the patient is taking, particularly valproate, lithium and serotonin re-uptake inhibitors.

- **Intention tremor with minimal or no postural tremor** (cerebellar dysfunction). Look for confirmatory signs of cerebellar dysfunction such as nystagmus, dysarthria, dysmetria, dyssynergia, dysdiadochokinesia, loss of check and wide-based unsteady gait, and other evidence of ataxia. It is important not to confuse this tremor, which *only* appears as the hand or foot approaches its target during the finger-to-nose or the toe-to-finger manoeuvre ('terminal tremor'), with a kinetic tremor ('dynamic tremor'). The latter is present in patients with essential tremor, along with the more typical postural tremor, but patients with essential tremor usually do not have overt signs of ataxia except for difficulties with tandem gait.

Other signs of cerebellar dysfunction:

Eye movement abnormalities (see Chapter 9):
- Jerky pursuit
- Gaze-evoked nystagmus
- Square wave jerks

Dysarthria. Slurred or scanning ('robotic') speech (see Chapter 12)

Overshoot (dysmetria)
- Loss of check. This is one of the most characteristic signs of cerebellar dysfunction. It is manifested by the inability of the patient to stop a rapidly moving limb, often associated with 'rebound', or an overshoot followed by an exaggerated movement in the opposite direction. There are two ways to elicit the sign. First, the patient is asked to raise his or her extended arms above the head and then instructed to rapidly lower the arms into a horizontal position. A patient with a unilateral cerebellar lesion will continue to move the ipsilateral arm below the horizontal position ('loss of check') and then often overcorrects by moving the arm above the horizontal position ('rebound'). Another way to elicit 'loss of check' is to ask patients to forcefully flex their elbows against the examiner's hand. When the examiner suddenly removes the hand, the patient with a cerebellar lesion will continue to flex the elbow and, if unprotected, could hit his own face. It is, therefore, very important to always protect the patient's face during this manoeuvre.

Dysrhythmia. Here the patient has difficulty sustaining a simple rhythm in, for example, patting the thigh with one hand.

Wide-based unsteady gait (see Chapter 6).

- **Other tremors**
  - *Dystonia tremor syndromes.* Patients with dystonia, such as cervical dystonia (e.g. torticollis) or hand dystonia often have an associated tremor. This so-called

dystonic tremor has the same distribution as the dystonia (head or hand, respectively, in the examples listed) and is manifested by irregular tremor that increases in amplitude as the patient tries to resist the abnormal pulling and may stop completely when the affected body part is allowed to assume the position to which it is pulled, the so-called null point. Patients with dystonia often also have a tremor in the body part otherwise unaffected by the dystonia. Thus, a patient with torticollis may have a marked tremor of the outstretched hands. Look for obvious dystonic posturing of the neck or upper limbs (e.g. splaying of the fingers with deviation of the wrist or shoulders). Many patients have subtle findings of abnormal posturing, and it may be unclear where such patients sit in the dystonic tremor syndrome-essential tremor spectrum. Such tremors are currently described as 'essential tremor plus'.[1]

- *Holmes (rubral, midbrain or cerebellar outflow) tremor.* This is a coarse, often proximal, tremor of the upper limb which may be present at rest, but which increases in amplitude with the arms outstretched and is maximal when approaching a target ('terminal tremor'). It used to be called a 'rubral tremor' on the basis that it arose from the red nucleus of the midbrain, but this is no longer thought to be the case and it has been renamed the Holmes tremor after Gordon Holmes who wrote the definitive description of it. The presence of a contralateral oculomotor palsy in some cases points to the midbrain as the likely site of the lesion causing this tremor. The combination of cerebellar outflow tremor with or without ipsilateral hemiparesis and contralateral oculomotor palsy is referred to as the Benedict syndrome.

 See Video 60 Holmes tremor
Coarse postural and intention tremor in a patient with midbrain lesion.

- **Wing-beating tremor.** This refers to a striking, coarse tremor involving the proximal muscles of the upper limb. It can be seen in essential tremor, dystonic tremor syndromes and parkinsonian tremor, but when this is seen in a young adult, you should think of Wilson's disease.[1] Carefully inspect the cornea, illuminated from the side with your flashlight, for the characteristic brown rings (like a brown arcus senilis) described by Kayser[2] and Fleischer.[3]

1. SA Kinnear Wilson, Queen Square neurologist (1874–1937).
2. Bernard Kayser, German ophthalmologist (1869–1954).
3. Richard Fleischer, German physician (1848–1909).

 See Video 61 Bat's wing tremor in a patient with Wilson's disease

At rest, he has a head tremor (titubation); with the arms abducted at the shoulder and flexed at the elbow, he develops a coarse asymmetrical proximal tremor of the arms.

See Video 62 Slow tremor

Slow tremor (myorhythmia) in a patient with Wilson's disease.

Box 10.1   Tips

● If you are wondering whether or not the patient has Parkinson's disease, get them to walk. Patients with Parkinson's disease nearly always fail to swing one or both arms fully. One exception to this is a patient who is so responsive to levodopa, that, while the drug is working, all signs of the disease disappear. Other characteristic features to observe are a slow, shuffling gait, intermittent freezing, particularly when walking through narrow passages such as the doorway, and turning en bloc. There are, of course, a number of atypical parkinsonian syndromes – including progressive supranuclear palsy and multiple system atrophy (MSA) – which are manifested by gait and balance difficulties, but in contrast to Parkinson's disease, these abnormalities occur relatively early in their course.

 See Video 63 Progressive multiple system atrophy

Progressive MSA manifested by severe bradykinesia, dysarthria, dysautonomia with orthostatic hypotension, respiratory, gastrointestinal and urinary failure and marked sialorrhoea, precipitated by eating chocolate.

● If you wish to enhance a resting or postural tremor, in order to observe its characteristics more easily, ask the patient to subtract 7 from 100 and go on subtracting 7s as fast as possible, or say the months of the year backwards. The stress involved in doing this is guaranteed to increase the tremor. Parkinson's tremor is also exacerbated during walking.

● Chorea, most types of myoclonus and tics differ from tremor in one major way. They are not rhythmical (regular in their timing).

● In Parkinson's disease, the amplitude of the tremor is often more marked in one hand than in the other.

● The tremor in essential tremor, while maximal on holding the arms out, persists during movement and often increases as the finger approaches the target (e.g. the nose).

● Isolated head tremor is never due to Parkinson's disease, but may be seen in essential tremor, cervical dystonia (dystonic tremor), and cerebellar pathology (titurbation).

Other abnormal involuntary movements

Inspection 83

The movement 83

Drug-induced movement disorders 92

Abnormal involuntary movements can be relatively easy to recognize if you have seen such a case before (pattern recognition). All is not lost if you have not, for more important than jumping to conclusions is your ability to carefully and accurately describe what you see and then, based on the observed phenomenology, come up with a reasonable differential diagnosis.

Inspection

As always, step back and look at the patient as a whole. You have a number of questions in your mind:

● Which parts of the body are involved in the movements (focal, segmental, hemi-, generalized, symmetrical, asymmetrical)?

● What is the patient's posture (head, trunk, limbs)?

● What happens to the movements as the patient talks to you? Do they increase or lessen?

● Is the patient relating normally to you?

The movement

In choosing the most appropriate term to describe the movement, it is useful to start off with a general category that does not commit you to a particular diagnosis. Broadly categorize it as rhythmical (e.g. tremor, segmental myoclonus) or irregular (e.g. dystonic tremor, chorea, tics), jerk-like (e.g. myoclonus, chorea, tics) or sustained and patterned (e.g. dystonia).

DOI: 10.1201/9781003119166-11

● **Chorea.** The hallmark of chorea is random, twitchy movements that affect different parts of the body. In addition to the continuous movements of the limbs and trunk, chorea may be manifested by dancing of the eyebrows due to irregular contractions of the frontalis muscles. The movements often continue during standing and walking. Viewed as a whole, the patient with chorea appears to be in constant motion, restless, as you or I might be waiting for a bus with a full bladder. Yet, they usually do not feel restless and may not even be aware of the movements. Chorea can be generalized or confined to one side of the body (hemichorea). Chorea increases when the patient is talking or moving. There is often associated motor impersistence, such as milk-maid's grip and darting tongue (inability to sustain protrusion). There are many causes of chorea, including drugs (neuroleptics and levodopa), Huntington's disease and other genetic disorders, auto-immune disease such as systemic lupus

See Video 65 Sudden onset of mild left hemiparesis and marked left hemichorea- hemiballismus in a woman with new-onset diabetes mellitus
Brain CT scan and magnetic resonance imaging showed T1W, T2W and diffusion weighted imaging lesions in the right putamen and caudate, consistent with hyperglycaemia-induced hemichorea-hemiballismus. The involuntary movement is almost completely resolved with tetrabenazine, a monoamine-depleting drug.

● **Hemiballismus.** This is a violent, flinging or thrusting movement of the proximal arm and leg that occurs in random directions. So troublesome are the movements in some cases that the patient may sit on the hands to suppress them. The movements are of large amplitude but may be mixed with choreiform movements, into which hemiballismus often evolves over days to weeks. This movement disorder usually comes on quite suddenly, often following a stroke involving the contralateral subthalamic nucleus or its connections.

See Video 66 Hemiballismus
There are almost continuous irregular coarse jerks of the proximal part of the left arm which persist/increase during hand movement and walking.

● **Tics**. Motor tics most commonly involve the face and head, causing characteristic blinks, grimaces, poutings and head turns, but in some cases of Tourette's syndrome, the whole body may be affected with violent jerks or complex, sequential movements. The movements tend to lessen with distraction – for example, while talking – but they are voluntarily suppressed only with great difficulty. In addition to motor tics, patients with Tourette's syndrome also exhibit phonic tics, such as sniffing, grunting, squeaking and coughing. Sometimes, the involuntary sound resembles a loud bark or may present as a sudden scream. About 20 per cent of patients shout obscenities (swear words with sexual or racial connotation) or profanities (religious connotation), so-called coprolalia. This is often slipped in mid-sentence (like a tic, which of course it is) rather than delivered with the emphasis that is usually given to swearing. Obscene gestures (copropraxia) also commonly occur in the setting of Tourette's syndrome. One characteristic feature of tics, which helps differentiate this movement from other jerk-like movements, such as chorea or myoclonus, is the presence of a premonitory sensation that can occur in a crescendo before or during a tic or as a more generalized urge to make the movement or sound. Patients often describe a need to make the movement and experience a sense of relief after its execution. Many patients with Tourette's syndrome also have obsessive-compulsive disorder and attention deficit disorder with or without hyperactivity. Although the majority of children with Tourette's syndrome experience marked improvement or spontaneous remission in their tics by the time they reach their 20s, tics can persist into adulthood or can recur later in life.

 See Video 67 Tourette's syndrome
Blinking, grimacing and platysma contraction are seen, particularly when the patient talks.

 See Video 68 Severe Tourette's syndrome
Severe Tourette's syndrome manifested by complex motor and blocking tics, as well as phonic tics associated with marked obsessive-compulsive disorder and self-injurious behaviour.

● **Myoclonus.** This refers to sudden brief, shock-like, muscle twitches which can affect any part of the body. Depending on the setting, they may occur spontaneously or only in response to a stimulus such as a noise, visual threat, touch or pinprick (stimulus-sensitive myoclonus). Myoclonus often increases with voluntary movement (action or intention myoclonus). In some cases, the twitches are time-locked to an electroencephalography (EEG) event and may be regarded as a 'fragment' of an epileptic seizure. The movement is usually associated with a muscular contraction, but it can also be caused by gravity as the muscle momentarily loses tone. This is known as '**negative myoclonus**' or, more commonly, '**asterixis**' (or in the setting of hepatic failure, '**liver flap**').

 See Video 69 Reflex myoclonus
Flicking the fingers of the right hand makes the arm jump. Pricking the fingers causes an exaggerated withdrawal reflex.

 See Video 70 Post-hypoxic myoclonus
At rest, this patient is still, but when she raises her arms or legs, large-amplitude, shock-like jerks are seen. The jerks interfere with her attempt to touch a pointer, but there is no true intention tremor.

 See Video 71 Asterixis
The outstretched hands and fingers repeatedly drop and then recover, reflecting a momentary loss of tone.

In hospital practice, myoclonus is seen most commonly in the setting of metabolic disturbance, such as renal or hepatic encephalopathy, diabetic ketoacidosis, post-hypoxic brain injury, epileptic syndromes and degenerative disease of the brain (e.g. MSA). The site of origin of myoclonus determines, to some extent, its clinical features:

- *Cortical myoclonus:* low-amplitude, irregular twitches of individual fingers or the upper limb, induced by voluntary movement and sometimes touch, sudden perturbation or pinprick and associated with giant somatosensory evoked potentials (SSEPs).

See Video 72 Mini-myoclonus
There are fine, shock-like lateral movements of individual fingers.

- *Brainstem myoclonus:* generalized jerks, often of the neck, shoulders and proximal limbs and sometimes the facial or bulbar musculature, often triggered by noise or other stimuli.

See Video 73 Palatal and laryngeal myoclonus

- *Spinal myoclonus:* slow (about 1–2 Hz), rhythmical jerks of the trunk or limbs, often involving just a few adjacent spinal segments.
- *Dystonia.* In dystonia, body parts are pulled into odd *postures* due to abnormal contraction of opposing sets of muscles. In addition to abnormal postures, *dystonia* is often manifested by superimposed jerky movements which may be regular (*dystonic tremor*) or irregular (*dystonic movements*). Dystonia may be *generalized* (involving the trunk and legs), *segmental* (involving two adjacent segments such as head and neck in cranial-cervical dystonia) or *focal* (e.g. blepharospasm, torticollis). It is usually induced or made worse by voluntary movement and in some cases only appears with specific activities (e.g. writer's cramp). A key feature in many cases is the presence of a geste antagonistique ('sensory trick'), whereby, for example, the

head posture of a patient with torticollis improves if the patient touches the cheek. (Interestingly, the correction may occur before the hand reaches the face.) Dystonia is often only mild-moderately disabling, confined to use of the affected body part; in rare instances, it can be generalised and life-threatening (so-called status dystonius or dystonic storm). In some families, dystonia and myoclonus occur together. Rarely, dystonia can occur in paroxysms, either triggered by voluntary movement (paroxysmal kinesigenic or exertional dyskinesia) or occurring out of a background of rest or normal activity (paroxysmal non-kinesigenic dyskinesia). Task-specific dystonia occurs mainly or only with certain activities.

 See Video 74 Athetosis

The fingers of the outstretched right hand make continuous writhing slow irregular movements, each finger moving independently. Similar, low-amplitude movements are seen in the face involving the mouth, eyelids and eyebrows.

 See Video 75 Generalized dystonia

The patient's head is turned to the right and the mouth pulls to the left as he talks. The fingers of the left hand are splayed, and the left elbow and wrist are flexed. All actions are interrupted by slow involuntary movements of his limbs and neck.

 See Video 76 Torticollis

The head is turned to the left and tilted to the right. The posture is corrected by touching the cheeks with either hand (even before the hand touches): geste antagonistique. Even imagining the geste temporarily corrects the posture.

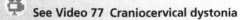 **See Video 77 Craniocervical dystonia**

Craniocervical dystonia and dystonic-respiratory dysregulation.

 **See Video 78 Myoclonus-dystonia syndrome**

Myoclonus-dystonia syndrome secondary to mutation in the gene coding for ε-sarcoglycan.

 **See Video 79 Paroxysmal kinesigenic dystonia**

 **See Video 80 Task-specific dystonia**

Task-specific dystonia in a professional violinist manifested by involuntary left fifth finger flexion and compensatory extension.

- Blepharospasm must be distinguished from apraxia of eyelid opening, where the eyes are not usually 'screwed up' due to forceful contraction of the orbicularis oculi, but instead, the patient has trouble opening the eyes after they are closed.

See Video 81 Apraxia of eyelid opening
Marked apraxia of eyelid opening

- **Athetosis.** This comprises slow, writhing, irregular dystonic movements of individual fingers and toes, and other parts of the limbs and sometimes the face, typically occurring in the setting of cerebral palsy.

- **Stereotypies.** These are repetitive movements, such as arm flapping, which can be normal in children but which are more marked and persistent in disorders such as autism.

See Video 82 Stereotypies
Marked stereotypies associated with Rett syndrome.

See Video 83 Stereotypic behaviour: repeatedly pushing a button on a remote control and foot and finger tapping in a right-handed man with progressive dysarthria, apathy, anxiety and mouth drooling
His hand-face stereotypies markedly improved with tetrabenazine, a monoamine-depleting drug.

See Video 84 Dopa-induced, peak-dose dyskinesia
The head tilts initially to the right and then the left. While seated, the patient's legs and feet move restlessly. While walking, the head tilts to the right, and the fingers of the left hand writhe and posture.

See Video 85 Chorea in Huntington's disease
This patient makes constant twitching movements of her hands and feet; she grimaces and her eyebrows dance. All this increases when she talks.

See Video 67 Tourette's syndrome

See Video 72 Mini-myoclonus

See Video 75 Generalized dystonia

See Video 76 Torticollis

See Video 86 Blepharospasm/cranial dystonia
The eyes keep screwing up, and there are 'rabbit twitches' of the nose and upper lip.

Drug-induced movement disorders

Having been through the diagnostic process as described, there remains a group of conditions which do not fit readily into the aforementioned schema. These are the drug-induced movement disorders. They are more common than most of the conditions considered so far, and in some cases preventable, and for these reasons deserve special consideration.

● **Dopa-induced involuntary movements**. Most patients with Parkinson's disease who respond to levodopa eventually develop involuntary movements related to the drug regimen. This problem occurs earlier in younger-onset patients. There are two main types:

- *Peak-dose dyskinesia*. About an hour after taking a dose, the patient starts to make choreo-ballistic or choreo-dystonic movements which may be maximal in the limbs, face, neck or trunk. Often, the patient is unaware or untroubled by the movements. They last for an hour or two but are made worse by taking another dose of levodopa while they are still present.

See Video 84 Dopa-induced, peak-dose dyskinesia

- *Beginning and/or end-of-dose dystonia*. This occurs as the benefit from a dose of levodopa wears off, or in the early morning before the first dose, and comprises a painful cramping of the toes which makes walking difficult. It is relieved by taking another dose of levodopa.

See Video 87 End-of-dose dystonia
The patient has a stiff upright posture with no arm swing, walking on the outside of the left foot, with the hallux dorsiflexed.

- **Tardive syndromes**. Nearly every known movement disorder can be encountered as a result of acute or chronic exposure to drugs, such as dopamine-receptor blocking drugs (neuroleptics) and many other drugs. While the classic neuroleptic drugs prescribed for various psychiatric conditions, such as trifluoperazine, chlorpromazine and haloperidol, have been typically associated with tardive syndromes, anti-emetics, such as prochlorperazine and metoclopramide, can also do the same. Although the second- and third-generation neuroleptics have been thought to have a lower risk, all of them, with the possible exception of clozapine, can also cause tardive syndromes. Older patients, particularly women, are most prone to develop this drug-induced movement disorder. There are many different types of tardive dyskinesia, defined as any involuntary movement that develops during chronic drug exposure and which may persist or even be triggered following discontinuation of the offending dopamine-receptor blocking drug.

- *Akathisia*. This refers to a feeling of restlessness which is reflected in an inability to keep still for any length of time. The patient often paces the floor like a caged tiger. The movements themselves are stereotypic and are accompanied by a strong sensory component, an urge to move.

See Video 88 Tardive akathisia
The patient has continuous restless movements of the limbs and is unable to keep still. He also has tardive dyskinesia and repeatedly protrudes his tongue.

See Video 89 Akathisia
Akathisia induced by selective serotonin reuptake inhibitor.

- *Tardive dyskinesia*. This drug-induced movement disorder is characterized by continuous, stereotypic, movements of the mouth, tongue and jaw (buccolingual dyskinesia/oromandibular dystonia). They are often worse when the patient talks. In addition to orofacial movements, patients with tardive dyskinesia may have involvement of other body parts and may also complain of sensory phenomena, such as burning pain or other discomfort in the mouth or genital area. Paradoxically, the movements initially get worse when the offending drug is withdrawn and may persist for years thereafter.

See Video 90 Tardive dyskinesia
This patient continually pouts her lips, protrudes her tongue and closes her eyes.

See Video 91 Severe oromandibular dystonia with bruxism (constant grinding of the teeth) resulting in extensive dental damage
The symptoms were subsequently controlled with botulinum toxin injections into the masseter and temporalis muscles.

See Video 92 Tardive lingual dyskinesia (stereotypy)

See Video 77 Craniocervical dystonia

See Video 93 Typical tardive dyskinesia manifested by orofacial-lingual stereotypy

- *Tardive dystonia*. This is most commonly seen in young males treated with neuroleptics for schizophrenia. The typical posture is that of neck and trunk extension (retrocollis and opisthotonus) with arms extended and pronated. Again, the problem is made transiently worse by withdrawal of the drug which caused the problem.

See Video 94 Tardive dystonia

The neck and trunk are hyperextended, except when the patient clasps his hands behind his neck (geste antagonistique).

- *Drug-induced parkinsonism.* Neuroleptic drugs may produce a syndrome identical to idiopathic Parkinson's disease. This may persist for a year after the drugs are withdrawn.
- *Drug-induced tremors.* There are many drugs, such as lithium, valproate and serotonin-uptake inhibitors, that can cause tremors that may be phenomenologically similar to either parkinsonian or essential tremor.

Box 11.1   Tips

- With any involuntary movement, the first decision is whether the movement is rhythmical. If it is not rhythmical, it is better not to call it a tremor.
- The hallmark of chorea is that it is flitting and unpredictable (random).
- The key to understanding tics is the premonitory urge that the patient feels before the movement and relief when it is executed – Kinnear Wilson likened it to a sneeze.
- The essence of myoclonus is its 'shock-like' or 'jerk-like' quality, which may be stimulus-induced, such as a loud noise and sudden visual threat, but not preceded by a premonitory sensation.
- Dystonia is characterized by patterned, repetitive contractions of muscles causing abnormal movements and postures.

12 Language and speech disturbance

General approach 97
Dysarthria 99
Aphasia 100

Speech disturbance is usually one of two types: dysarthria or aphasia. When it is due to *dysarthria* – a problem of articulation – the patient will usually be acutely aware of the problem. With *aphasia* – a problem of language – the patient may not be aware of the problem or is unable to explain it. Dysarthria usually arises from impairment at a subcortical level of muscle control needed to speak clearly. Aphasia arises from impairment, usually at a cortical level, of the thinking processes which underly language. Aphasia usually arises from focal lesions involving the dominant cerebral hemisphere (usually the left, even in left-handed patients) of the brain. Language may also be impaired in dementia and many other neurodegenerative disorders where there is widespread disturbance of function in the cerebral hemispheres (see Chapter 13).

General approach

● Most patients with speech disturbance – particularly those with aphasia – find conversation an effort and easily become distressed. The exception is the patient with a severe Wernicke's (also known as a fluent or receptive) aphasia, who will speak fluently but nonsensically ('word salad') without insight. It is important to make the patient feel at ease. Do not stand over them; sit with them. If it is clear that they are struggling, reassure them that you appreciate how upsetting it is not to be able to communicate.

● Engage them in conversation on a topic with which they are likely to feel comfortable: 'Tell me about your job (family, holidays, hobbies, etc.)', or 'Describe the room around you in sentences'. Your wish is to hear the patient forming sentences, so avoid questions to which the answer is likely to be 'yes' or 'no'. It is often difficult to get a patient to speak freely. In this case, show them a picture (Figure 12.1) and ask them to describe the scene. This approach has the advantage that you can tell what the patient

DOI: 10.1201/9781003119166-12

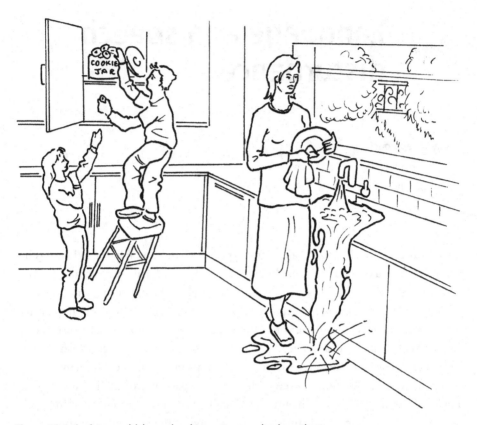

Figure 12.1 A picture which can be shown to an aphasic patient.

is trying to say (see the following). Do not rush this part of the examination, for it forms the basis of your assessment.

- The first thing to decide is whether you are dealing with dysarthria or aphasia. As the patient talks, pay particular attention to the following aspects of their speech:
  - Is the patient speaking with normal words and sentences which are simply slurred (not properly articulated)? You are dealing with a dysarthria.
  - Is the patient speaking with abnormal words and phrases or sentence structure? You are dealing with an aphasia.
  - Does the patient speak fluently (i.e. with normal speed and smoothly without inappropriate pauses), but the sentences have no real meaning? You are dealing with a fluent aphasia.
  - Does the patient speak hesitantly and effortfully or appear to have word-finding difficulties? You are dealing with a non-fluent aphasia.
  - Abnormal sentence structure, incorrect use of words or substitution of words close to the meaning or sound of appropriate words help confirm you are dealing with aphasia rather than dysarthria.

- Is there facial asymmetry? Is the right hand used as much as the left? A right hemiparesis often accompanies aphasia.

- Take note of the patient's 'body language'. Patients with non-fluent aphasia often have exaggerated body language. They sigh, gasp, roll their eyes and gesticulate, as they struggle to communicate with you. Sometimes they will burst into tears from sheer frustration. By contrast, patients who cannot communicate because of dementia may be unconcerned or unaware that there is a problem. Their body language is as impoverished as their speech.

Dealing with the two main patterns of abnormality, dysarthria and aphasia, in turn:

Dysarthria

Here, the words are slurred but the language content – if you were to write it down – is normal. The problem is one of articulation. Slurring of speech signifies weakness or incoordination of the muscles involved in the production of sounds. Common causes are spasticity (e.g. pseudobulbar palsy, MND), lower motor neurone bulbar weakness (e.g. progressive bulbar palsy, a form of MND) and cerebellar disorders (e.g. stroke or multiple sclerosis). With experience, one can confidently distinguish spastic from cerebellar dysarthria by the quality of speech. If you cannot, then you must rely on the neurological company which the dysarthria keeps.

Faint, quiet (dysphonic) speech is a feature of Parkinson's disease. The voice is also monotonous, and the words tend to run into each other. Weakness of the diaphragm and of other respiratory muscles also causes the voice to be low in volume.

Assessment of dysarthria involves five steps:

- *Repetition of words or phrases* which are difficult to say. Examples of these include
  - artillery, constitution, monotonous, autobiography; and
  - no ifs, ands or buts.

  Sometimes, a simple word can be correctly articulated but difficulty is encountered as the complexity of the word is progressively increased:
  - Zip, zipper, zippering
  - Please, pleasing, pleasingly
  - City, citizen, citizenship

- *Repetition of sounds* which test the different muscles of articulation. Where there is weakness of the lips, the patient will have difficulty saying 'puh' or 'bah', of the tongue 'tuh' or 'lah' and of the palate 'kuh' or 'gah'.

- Ask the patient to *cough*. A hoarse cough is heard where there is paralysis of a vocal cord due to a recurrent laryngeal nerve palsy.

- Examination of the motor system, in order to determine whether the problem is due to
  - a lower motor neurone lesion of the muscles of articulation (check for facial weakness; wasting, weakness or fasciculation of the tongue; loss of the gag reflex; or palatal palsy);
  - an upper motor neurone lesion of the muscles of articulation (brisk jaw jerk, exaggerated gag reflex, hemiparesis);
  - a cerebellar disturbance (nystagmus, intention tremor of the arms, gait disturbance); or
  - a hypokinetic dysarthria is typically seen in patients with Parkinson's disease, whereas hyperkinetic dysarthria is usually encountered in patients with involuntary movement disorders.
- Assessment of speech to determine whether patient has a language problem (aphasia) or slurring of speech (dysarthria), in which case the sentence structure, repetition and comprehension are usually normal (see the following discussion).

Aphasia

This refers to a disturbance in the production or understanding of language. The deficit usually applies to both spoken and written language but can occasionally be confined to one but not the other. Aphasia occurs with pathology of the dominant cerebral hemisphere. The main areas of the brain involved in language are shown in Figure 12.2. As a general rule, lesions of the frontal lobe ('anterior lesions') cause a non-fluent aphasia with preservation of comprehension. Other terms used for non-fluent aphasia include Broca's, 'expressive' or 'motor' aphasia. Lesions of the parietal and temporal lobes ('posterior lesions') cause a fluent aphasia, and there is impairment of comprehension. Other terms used for fluent aphasia include Wernicke's, 'receptive' or 'sensory' aphasia. Assessment of aphasia involves three steps.

1. Is the speech fluent or non-fluent?

   In a **non-fluent aphasia**, the patient's speech is effortful. Word approximations (semantic paraphasias, e.g. 'clock' instead of 'watch') or use of completely wrong words usually occur and may also be slurred. Sentences are short and lack 'filler' words such as 'and', 'the', 'so' and 'to'. The information content is often high. If you write down what is said, the result looks like a telegram – for example, 'Come hospital get better'. The normal melody (prosody) of speech is lost, and the patient often appears to be making an exaggerated effort to get the words out.

See Video 64 (see Chapter 11) Non-fluent aphasia following intracerebral haemorrhage from a left hemisphere arteriovenous malformation (AVM)
The patient exerts great effort to get any words out, and there are long pauses during which he gesticulates and appears to be frustrated; his sentences are short and easy to understand; his comprehension is normal.

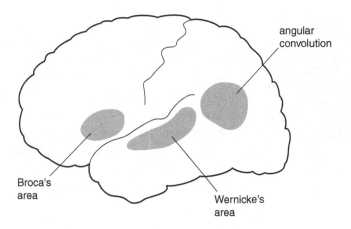

angular
convolution

Broca's
area

Wernicke's
area

Figure 12.2 The main language areas.

In a **fluent aphasia**, words flow freely, sentences are of a normal length, the voice rises and falls melodiously, but the information content is low. What is said is difficult to understand and words are used wrongly. When shown Figure 12.1, such a patient might say, 'The little boys and girls are getting up a stool and putting some cookies, right? Ah, this is the trouble the sing, the sing is overflowing, right?' Wrong words are known as paraphasias and are of three types:

- Phonemic or literal paraphasia, where a similar sounding but incorrect word is generated, e.g. a consonant may be substituted, causing the patient to say 'sing' when they mean 'sink'.
- Semantic paraphasia: a word is changed for another with an obvious association, e.g. a knife is called a fork.
- Neologism: a non-existent word is substituted for the intended word, e.g. a 'room' is called a 'boof'. Paraphasic errors usually signify involvement of the posterior speech areas except that phonemic/literal paraphasias may also occur in anterior aphasias. In mild cases, speech may be normal for a few sentences and then the sentence structure breaks down and paraphasias appear.

See Video 95 Wernicke's aphasia following a cardioembolic stroke
The patient speaks freely, but what he says is so littered with paraphasias as to make it almost impossible to understand. His comprehension is poor.

See Video 96 Fluent aphasia in a man with a left parietal glioma
He speaks freely with well-formed sentences and normal prosody (melody), at times making no mistakes; he then gets stuck 'and then for an extent for a week I was a problem with poising … voicing'. He appears to understand what is said to him but has great difficulty identifying and touching parts of his face in sequence. He is unable to repeat. In summary, he has a fluent aphasia with impaired comprehension and repetition, and he makes paraphasic errors.

2. Is the patient able to repeat?
   Patients with aphasia often have difficulty repeating the phrase 'no ifs, ands or buts'. They will say 'no ands or buts' or 'no ifs and buts', but never the full phrase. Words which are readily linked to a visual image, such as house, ship, book, face and cigarettes, can often be repeated without difficulty. It is thought that the memory stores of these words have a wider distribution within the brain than non-picture words, and are therefore less likely to be affected by lesions confined to the speech area. The inability to repeat is used in some classifications of aphasia which attempt to relate the type of aphasia with the site of the lesion. In practice, the main value of testing repetition is in confirming that the patient is aphasic.

3. Does the patient have normal comprehension?
   Patients with severe disturbance of comprehension often give the appearance that they fully understand everything that is said to them and, indeed, may think that they do understand. They smile or nod when there is a pause in the conversation. They gesticulate so convincingly that their problem may initially go unnoticed by their own family. These patients have normal body language, taking their cues from the movements of those around them and responding appropriately. In testing their comprehension, one must make allowance for the fact that they may not be able to

find the words to tell you that they understand what is being said to them. This is done in two ways:

- Reduce the amount of language that they need to use to the minimum: 'yes' or 'no'. Ask a sequence of questions: 'Are you in hospital?'; 'Are we sitting in your house?'; 'Have you got pyjamas on?'; 'Have you got a coat on?' Remember that the patient has an even chance, each time, of giving the correct response. Ask a number of questions, therefore, and vary them so that there are no sequences in which the same answer, 'yes' or 'no', would be correct. Perseveration is common in aphasia, causing the patient to repeat the same response several times. Subtle defects of comprehension may only be picked up by asking 'double-barrelled' questions: 'Do you put your shoes on before your socks?'; 'Do you put your socks on before your shoes?'; 'Do you shut the car door before getting into the car?'; 'If the lion ate the tiger, is the tiger alive?'

- Ask the patient to obey commands: 'Touch your nose', or 'Touch your knee'. Many patients with aphasia can obey single commands, but cannot follow sequences: 'Touch your chin, then your nose, then your ear'. Patients with normal comprehension are often unable to protrude the tongue on command due to an apraxia.

To summarize, in describing an aphasia you should state whether it was fluent or non-fluent, whether there were paraphasic errors and whether repetition and comprehension were impaired. A description such as this is probably more useful than terms such as 'nominal aphasia' or 'Wernicke's aphasia', which mean different things to different people. If you wish to use these terms, Table 12.1 provides a guide to their current usage.

To complete the examination, one should ask the patient to read and to write. The information obtained from doing this is similar to that gained from listening to the speech. Patients with non-fluent aphasias have great difficulty writing at all – even with the left hand. Patients with fluent aphasia make paraphasic errors in their reading and writing.

Table 12.1 Current definitions of aphasia.[a]

Speech type	Repetition	Comprehension	Associated signs
Non-fluent			
Broca's[b] aphasia	Impaired/normal	Normal	Weakness R arm
Global aphasia	Impaired	Impaired	R hemiparesis
Fluent			
Wernicke's aphasia	Impaired	Impaired	Homonymous hemianopia
Conduction aphasia	Impaired	Normal	
Isolation aphasia	Normal	Impaired	
Nominal aphasia	Normal	Normal	

[a] After Geschwind MD. Aphasia. *N Engl J Med* 1971; 284: 654–656.

[b] Pierre-Paul Broca, French anatomist and surgeon (1824–1880).

Box 12.1   Tips

- The subdivisions of aphasia, outlined in Table 12.1, provide a useful approach to patients with speech and language problems, but many patients do not fit comfortably into this or any other system of classification. Thus, it is not uncommon for patients – for example, with a posterior lesion – to have marked poverty of speech, albeit well articulated.

- The left hemisphere is dominant for language in the majority of individuals, regardless of their handedness.

- A fluent aphasia, with normal comprehension and repetition (nominal aphasia), is characteristically seen in metabolic encephalopathies.

- Gerstmann's[1] syndrome (finger agnosia, agraphia, acalculia and right-left disorientation), although a favourite diagnosis of many trainees faced with a patient with aphasia, is relatively rare, and there is, of course, little point in testing for these features in a patient who has severely impaired comprehension.

- In children, aphasia is almost always non-fluent, regardless of the site of the lesion.

- How do you assess the quality of speech in a severely aphasic patient who is almost mute? Get the patient to count to ten, calling out the first few numbers with them and 'conducting' them through the remainder by hand signals, and using yes/no and multiple-choice questions.

- It is common for trainees to miss impairment of comprehension through inadequate testing. They will hurriedly ask the patient to point out different body parts (hand, foot, elbow) while looking at the part in question. This may give the patient who is relying solely on body language all the help they need to perform the task.

1. Josef Gerstmann, Austrian neuropsychiatrist (1887–1969).

13 Higher cortical function testing

General approach 105
Formal cognitive testing 109
Some syndromes of dementia 110

Patients presenting for the first time with dementia often have little insight into their problem and it is the relatives who make the appointment or bring them to you. You will make the diagnosis mainly from the history that the relatives provide, but the neurological examination is important for confirming this.

General approach

As with the aphasic patient, your approach to the patient with cognitive impairment will make allowance for the fact that there are problems with communication and the patient is anxious or alarmed. Sit beside the patient and make every effort by your manner to put them at their ease. If the answers they give are to questions you didn't ask, be patient and resist the temptation to be hectoring in your efforts to gain more information. Better still, have a relative or friend present who can provide moral support and fill in the aspects of the history which the patient is unable to provide; patients with dementia often lack insight into their problem.

● **Delirium versus dementia**. One of your first tasks is to determine whether this is an acute potentially reversible problem of delirium or a longer-term problem of dementia. Of course, the patient may have both: patients with dementia are more prone to delirium if they develop, for example, an infection. The key to recognizing delirium is that it is characterized by fluctuations in attention, level of consciousness and/or confusion. As you begin to examine the patient, make note of certain key findings:
  - *Grooming*: if the patient is unkempt with long unwashed hair and decayed teeth, the problem is likely to be long-standing, in keeping with a history of dementia.
  - *Bruising*: note any facial bruising or black eyes, feel over the scalp for boggy swelling (over a skull fracture) and look behind the ears for the tell-tale bruising of Battle's sign (base of skull fracture). Any evidence of head trauma will encourage you to

DOI: 10.1201/9781003119166-13

perform the CT scan of the head earlier rather than later; you do not want to delay diagnosing a subdural haematoma.

- *Pulse, blood pressure, respiration.* Sweating, tachycardia, swings in blood pressure and altered breathing patterns are all common in delirium.
- *Level of consciousness*: dementia itself is not a cause of drowsiness. If the patient keeps falling asleep or is hard to rouse, you are dealing with delirium, most commonly due to *drug or alcohol overdose*, *infection* or *metabolic disturbance*. Delirious patients may go through periods of arousal in which they shout, moan or become aggressive. At these times, they may pluck restlessly at the sheets.
- *Attention.* Patients with delirium have a deficit in their ability to maintain attention, even if their level of consciousness is normal. After establishing the initial attention and trust of the patient, this can be tested by asking the patient to tap their hand the same number of one to three times every time the examiner taps their hand or asking the patient to count forwards out loud until the examiner says stop, and ensuring they can maintain the task for at least 30-60 s. More complex tests of higher function cannot be reliably assessed if the patient is inattentive – i.e. has a delirium. A delirium may also affect language processing.
- *Language.* In order to fully assess higher centres and cognition, language must also be intact and should be the first higher function tested after excluding delirium and establishing orientation. If the patient is aphasic, proceed to assess the patient's speech (Chapter 12). Aphasic patients may be mistakenly thought to have a delirium but should have a normal level of consciousness and attention.

● **Behaviour:** patients with frontal dementia can be *disinhibited* and *impulsive* (orbitofrontal cortex) and/or exhibit *executive dysfunction* (poor planning), *abulia* (loss of will) and *apathy* (lack of feeling) (dorsolateral prefrontal cortex). They usually have no complaints and do not initiate conversation as they lack insight. They may sit or lie for much of the day doing nothing and showing neither pleasure nor frustration. They are orientated, particularly for surroundings, and their responses to your questions may be sensible and appropriate, leading you to the erroneous conclusion that there is not much wrong with them.

Such patients may show *environmental dependence*: they are unable to inhibit their innate or acquired responses to external stimuli. Exploratory behaviour with the hands and mouth (grasping and groping), visual fixation and following, using objects (utilization behaviour) and mimicry are behaviours which are controlled by the frontal lobes. When the frontal lobes are not functioning normally, such behaviours are exhibited indiscriminately. They can be readily tested:

- *Forced grasping and groping.* Hold your index and middle fingers in a vertical plane (i.e. not in a normal 'hand-shaking' posture) close to the patient's hand. When they see the hand, they will reach out and grasp it.

 See Video 97 Groping

The patient reaches out and grasps the hands which are offered to him (even though he has been asked not to) and is unable to let go. He also grasps with his feet.

 See Video 98 Frontotemporal dementia

Frontotemporal dementia and marked grasp and snout reflexes, as well as foot stereotypies.

- The *grasp reflex* is tested by sliding your index and middle fingers across the palm of the hand. This is sometimes distinguished from the traction reflex where you run your fingers along the length of the patient's fingers – from base to tip – again causing him or her to grasp them. The latter is said to induce the response by inducing a stretch reflex in the finger flexors and will be positive in a patient with hyperreflexia of the upper limbs and no frontal lobe dysfunction. In practice, they provide very similar information. If the patient grips your fingers, ask them not to. Often, this will inhibit the response, but when you repeat the manoeuvre a few moments later, or after distraction, the grasping returns. A similar response is seen if you approach the patient's mouth with your index finger (after apologizing for the intrusion); the mouth opens and the patient may move the head forward to grasp the finger.

 See Video 99 Mouth grasp

This patient flexes her head and opens her mouth to an approaching finger even when asked not to.

- Such patients may also have forced visual following; in contrast to their general lack of activity, their eyes follow you as you move around the room or bed. If you move your penlight in a circle in front of them, they will follow it, even when asked not to.

See Video 100 Forced visual following (visual grasping)

The patient follows the light with her eyes, even though it circles uncomfortably. She is unable to suppress the behaviour.

- *Utilization behaviour.* Offer the patient your own or a colleague's glasses. The normal response is one of surprise. Patients with frontal lobe disinhibition will put them on, and a second and even a third pair if they are offered. If you give them your stethoscope they may attempt to use it. These patients tend to fiddle endlessly with whatever catches their attention: dressing gown cord, bed head, sheets.

See Video 101 Utilization behaviour

The patient stacks three pairs of spectacles on his nose, one at a time, as each is offered to him.

- *Imitation behaviour (mimicry).* While conversing, put your arm out or up and hold it for a few seconds. The patient with frontal disinhibition will tend to copy you. This, incidentally, is not an aspect of the examination you will want to try on patients with normal cognition!

See Video 102 Forced mimicry

When the examiner raises his hand with two fingers extended, the patient incorporates the posture into his own gestures. He also imitates left arm raising, both arm raising, right fist clenching and left leg raising, while continuing the conversation.

Formal cognitive testing

After establishing that level of consciousness and attention are intact, each component of the formal cognitive examination is aimed at probing higher functions subserved by different lobes of the brain, in the same way that the routine neurological examination probes functions of lower levels of the nervous system.

Although modern theories of cerebral function focus on the role of widely distributed networks subserving different functions, the principle of different lobes of the brain having a major role in specific cognitive processes still holds, including the concept of the dominant versus non-dominant hemisphere.

As outlined in detail in Chapter 12, the dominant hemisphere, especially the frontotemporal lobes, is largely responsible for language and if damaged results in aphasia. If the patient is aphasic, acknowledge that this may limit interpretation of additional cognitive testing before proceeding. Next test dominant parietal lobe function by examining writing, calculation, left-right orientation and finger naming (a command such as 'touch your right ear with your left little finger' quickly tests the last two), deficits in which constitute Gertmann's syndrome (agraphia, acalculia, left-right disorientation and finger agnosia). The non-dominant parieto-occipital cortices have a major role in visuospatial function. Test for ability to copy a cube and draw a clock face, including putting in the numbers, to look for hemi-spatial neglect. Look for dressing apraxia by asking the patient to put on a cardigan or jacket which has been turned partly inside out. The left and right frontoparietal lobes also have a vital role in higher order control of learned motor functions such as tool use and gestures. Loss of higher order motor control results in a deficit known as apraxia. Ask the patient to imitate you making a couple of hand gestures such as a 'V' victory or 'OK' sign, demonstrate how they would salute or wave goodbye and demonstrate how they would use a pair of scissors which they were holding in their hand, looking for movements in the wrong plane or using the wrong movement or joints – e.g. 'hand as tool' The dominant and non-dominant temporal lobes, respectively, have a major role in encoding verbal and non-verbal (visuospatial) memory. Often at the bedside, only verbal memory is examined by testing delayed recall of a list of three to five words. Firstly, test immediate recall to ensure that working memory is intact. Visuospatial memory in formal neuropsychometric assessment is classically tested by asking a patient to reproduce a drawing of a meaningless diagram, the Rey complex figure. Finally, probe frontal lobe function. Ask the patient to perform a Luria three-step command, making in sequence a fist, cut, then palm action with each hand, looking for perseverative sequence errors indicative of frontal lobe dysfunction, but also motor gestural errors arising from apraxia. Examine for other evidence of frontal lobe dysfunction as described earlier. Evidence of frontal lobe dysfunction is best gained from the history given by the family: loss of insight, inappropriate behaviour, impairment of judgement in financial and personal matters and loss of the ability to organize home or work activities. These are difficult things for the non-expert to gauge, particularly when there are time constraints. The features of abulia and release of behaviours outlined earlier only become apparent in moderately advanced cases of frontal dementia.

For bedside quantification of cognitive function, the Mini-Mental State Examination (MMSE) is now used routinely in most hospitals. With its emphasis on orientation and memory (it was designed as a screening test for Alzheimer's disease[1]), it is not a sensitive test of frontal lobe function. The Montreal Cognitive Assessment (MoCA) is a more sensitive test as it includes items that examine frontal executive function. What follows is an abbreviated and modified version of the Addenbrooke's Cognitive Examination (Figure 13.1). This will provide you with a flavour of the sort of problems the patient may be experiencing in orientation, memory, verbal fluency, language and visuospatial sense.

Some syndromes of dementia

By definition, in dementia, there is progressive impairment of memory and deficits in at least one other cognitive domain (speech, praxis, executive function or visuospatial function) sufficient to produce occupational or social disability. The pattern of abnormality varies according to which part of the brain is affected:

- **Alzheimer's syndrome**
  - Initially, impairment of memory
  - Later extends to all other domains: spatial sense, language, frontal executive function

- **Dementia of frontal lobe type**
  - Initially, change in behaviour with loss of social skills, loss of verbal fluency
  - Later, loss of organizational skills, judgement
  - Eventually, abulia and frontal release behaviour
  - Three subtypes of frontal dementia are recognized:
    - Dorsolateral: executive dysfunction
    - Orbitofrontal: disinhibition
    - Medial: akinetic mutism

- **Dementia in parkinsonism**
  - This occurs only after many years of idiopathic Parkinson's disease when it causes slowing of thinking, spontaneous fluctuations of cognitive function over hours or days, visual hallucinations and paranoid delusions (often at night) with good preservation of social skills. One of the clues that the patient is developing cognitive impairment is the appearance of apraxia of the hands. They cannot accurately copy

---

1. Alois Alzheimer, German pathologist (1864–1915).

Selected Tests modified from the Addenbrooke's Cognitive Examination	*Patient's name* DOB MRN Date	
ORIENTATION Year? .... Month? .... Day of the week?	Country? .... State/County? .... Hospital? .... Floor?	
ANTEROGRADE MEMORY Repeat this name and address and flower Peter Marshall 42 Market St Newcastle Daffodil (Test recall after 5 minutes)	*RETROGRADE MEMORY* Name of PM? USA President? *ATTENTION* Say the months backwards	
LANGUAGE Ask the patient to: give the name for the hands of your watch, the sole of your shoe, the nib of your pen	Point to the door, floor and ceiling	Repeat 'No ifs, ands, or buts'
APRAXIA Ask the patient to mime holding a piece of paper with the left hand and to cut it with a pair of scissors in the right hand. If he/she makes scissoring movements with the index and middle fingers, remind him that he/she is holding the scissors. If he/she has difficulty, repeat with real paper and scissors		
VERBAL FLUENCY Tell me as many words as you can think of beginning with the letter P, but not people or places. You have one minute to go (> 9)	Tell me the names of as many animals as you can think of in 1 minute, beginning with any letter of the alphabet (> 17)	
VISUOSPATIAL ABILITIES Ask the patient to copy your drawing of a cube	Draw a circle and ask the patient to fill in the numbers of the clock	

Figure 13.1 Modified version of the Addenbrooke's Cognitive Examination.

the movement you demonstrate to test bradykinesia. They cannot copy you when you make a fist, cut and palm motion with one hand on the other (Luria's test).[2] They cannot mime slicing a loaf of bread with a knife or cutting a piece of paper with a pair of scissors without using the hand as the tool (even when corrected) or making errors in the sequence of movements or position that the limbs adopt.

See Video 103 Apraxia in Parkinson's disease
This patient is unable to copy accurately the akinesia test for Parkinsonism, flexing the interphalangeal joints, as well as the metacarpophalangeal joints.

See Video 104 Luria test
The patient is not able to follow the sequence of fist, cut and slap.

See Video 105 Miming in apraxia
The patient is able to obey a simple sequence of pointing commands (showing that her comprehension is reasonable) but is unable to mime cutting a loaf.

- Dementia with Lewy bodies. In contrast to Parkinson's disease dementia, where cognitive decline occurs in the latter stages of the disease, patients with dementia with Lewy bodies often have cognitive decline, mental fluctuations and, most characteristically, visual hallucinations even before the onset of motor parkinsonian features.
- Dementia of frontal lobe type is prominent in progressive supranuclear palsy (PSP), although it may not be apparent until the latter stages of the disease.

---

2. Aleksander Romanovich Luria, Russian aphasiologist (1902–1977).

● **Vascular dementia**
  • This is characterized by lower half parkinsonism, affecting mainly the legs with a broad-based shuffling gait, often with preserved arm swing in contrast to Parkinson's disease, occurring on a background of hypertension and other stroke risk factors. The course may have a stepwise progression, and the examination may also reveal emotional lability and brisk jaw and other reflexes.

● **Creutzfeldt–Jakob disease**
  • This is a rare cause of dementia which has to be considered when the patient deteriorates over weeks and months rather than years and has prominent myoclonic jerks.

 See Video 106 Creutzfeldt–Jakob disease
Rapidly progressive cognitive decline, apraxia, ataxia, myoclonus and spasticity secondary to Creutzfeldt–Jakob disease.

Box 13.1   Tips

● If a confused patient is drowsy, the immediate problem is likely to be one of delirium, probably caused by some metabolic encephalopathy.

● The most useful aspect of the clinical assessment is the history obtained from the patient's relatives or spouse.

● The MMSE does not adequately test frontal lobe function. The MoCA is a better short bedside tool.

● The earliest feature of frontal lobe dysfunction which is readily tested is impairment of verbal fluency (generation of words).

● Signs of advanced frontal lobe dysfunction include abulia, grasping and groping, utilization behaviour and forced mimicry.

● The patient who is worried that he/she might have Alzheimer's disease rarely does: loss of insight is an early feature of dementia in Alzheimer's disease.

● Always run through the checklist of reversible dementias:
  • 'Pseudo-dementia' due to depression
  • Hypothyroidism
  • Vitamin B$_{12}$ deficiency
  • Frontal meningioma
  • Normal pressure hydrocephalus

● When discussing memory, the old classification of short- and long-term memory loss is no longer adequate. You should become familiar with the following terms:
  - *Declarative memory:* all the facts that you are able to recall, comprising the following:
    - *Episodic (autobiographical) memory:* events in your own life linked to a specific time and place.
    - *Semantic memory:* the body of general knowledge, linguistic skills and vocabulary which you have acquired.
  - *Procedural memory:* the memory of motor skills you have acquired.
  - *Working memory:* the ability to retain the information necessary to complete a task or to hold a conversation.

14 Assessment of coma

The Glasgow coma scale 118
Some distinctive types of coma 118

Patients who are drowsy or comatose pose a particular problem, as so much of the routine neurological examination relies on the ability of the patient to cooperate and follow instructions. A different approach is therefore required. Often the patient is already intubated, ventilated, sedated and even paralysed by the time you get the opportunity to examine them, and some drugs may need to be temporarily withdrawn or reversed, under certain circumstances, to perform the neurological examination.

Coma results from impaired function of the brainstem reticular formation. The most common cause is drug overdose, but other causes include severe head injury, hypoxic brain injury, infections (like bacterial meningitis or viral encephalitis) metabolic disturbance like diabetic coma or hepatic failure, subarachnoid haemorrhage, exposure to toxins (e.g. carbon monoxide), encephalitis and severe raised intracranial pressure.

Lesions of the cerebral hemisphere do not cause coma unless they are very extensive and impinge, usually by mass effect, on brainstem function.

Watch what you say when speaking at the bedside with colleagues, staff and relatives. Never assume the patient is not listening – they may be 'locked in' (see below).

The role of the neurological examination in coma is to assess its level so that changes may be documented and to determine which parts of the central nervous system (in particular, the brainstem and cerebral hemispheres) are still functioning. In deep coma, the question may arise as to whether brain death has occurred.

What follows is a list of examination techniques used in assessing coma. In the setting of the emergency situation, the immediate issues concern whether the patient

● has an adequate airway;

● is breathing normally or has Cheyne-Stokes (waxing and waning) breathing, hyperpnoea or hypopnoea;

● has adequate blood pressure and circulatory perfusion;

● smells of acetone (diabetic coma) or alcohol or other toxic substances;

DOI: 10.1201/9781003119166-14

- has jaundice, cyanosis or pallor;

- has life-threatening issues, such as internal or external bleeding or major bony injuries (including the possibility of spinal injury if there has been trauma); or

- has signs of infection – check temperature and pulse rate.

Once these are attended to, attention can be directed to an examination of the nervous system:

- **Pupils**. One of the first questions to answer is whether coma is due to a toxic/metabolic cause or due to intracranial pathology. The pupils provide a major clue. Are the pupils of a normal size for the degree of illumination in the room, symmetrical and responsive to light? In coma, due to toxic metabolic causes, the pupils are usually normal; pin-point pupils may be due to opiate overdose, which must always be excluded. Focal intracranial pathology causes pupillary abnormalities; always exclude hypoglycaemia which can cause focal neurological signs, and ensure fixed dilated pupils are not due to applications of eye drops for an eye examination.

- **Inspection**. The posture of the patient is noted, including asymmetry of the head or limbs. Are there spontaneous movements of the head or limbs, and are they symmetrical? Are the eyes closed? Spontaneous blinking suggests that the pontine reticular formation is functioning. Is there bruising, particularly around the orbits or behind the ears (skull fracture)? Is there a boggy swelling on the scalp (skull fracture)?

- **Level of awareness**. Does the patient obey verbal commands? This test of cerebral hemisphere function may seem unnecessary in a patient who appears to be comatose but occasionally it turns out that they are 'locked in'; their cerebral hemispheres are functioning normally, they are fully conscious but they cannot make any movements apart from raising and lowering their eyes. The lesion is in the pons. Ask them to try to look up and down.

- **Fundi**. Look for papilledema (raised intracranial pressure) and subhyaloid haemorrhages (subarachnoid haemorrhage).

- **Doll's eye movements (oculocephalic reflex)**. This is not something that can be done when the patient is first admitted as it is essential to establish first that there has been no neck injury or arterial dissection in the neck. This test is most useful later in the course of the admission to test brainstem function, particularly if brain death is a consideration. Roll the head briskly from side to side, pausing briefly at the end of each movement and observe whether the eyes, which you are holding open, remain stationary (which means they have rotated in the opposite direction). This indicates an intact oculocephalic reflex which requires intact upper brainstem function. Flexing and extending the neck will similarly induce reflex vertical eye movements. Doll's eye movements are also usually preserved in metabolic coma. A patient with intact consciousness can also suppress their oculocephalic reflex.

- **Corneal reflex**. Touch the corneas in turn with cotton wool to see if the patient blinks and if the eyes roll up (Bell's phenomenon). If they do, the pathways between the midbrain Vth n. nuclei) and lower pons (VIIth n. nuclei) are intact.

- **Nose tickle**. Insert a piece of cotton wool into each nostril in turn and look for grimacing and limb movements. This is a neglected but most useful test. In a light coma, the patient will reach up and rub their nose. If there is a hemiparesis, only one hand will do this. If there is hemianaesthesia, tickling only one nostril will induce a response.

- **Cough reflex**. In an intubated patient, the cough reflex may be tested by suctioning with a catheter.

- **Gag reflex**. This is also not something that should be done in the initial assessment, as it may induce vomiting and inhalation of vomitus. It is mostly used after the patient has been intubated and one is testing brainstem function, particularly when brain death is a consideration. Touch the back of the throat alternately, left and right sides with similar pressure, with a cotton-tipped probe, while the tongue is depressed with a wooden tongue depressor.

- Tone of neck and limbs

- Jaw jerk

- Limb reflexes

- Plantar responses

- Response to painful stimuli
  - Squeeze the pectoralis muscles firmly on each side and press the nail beds of digits gently in all four limbs in turn with the handle of your tendon hammer. Several types of responses may be observed. The normal response is to push the stimulus away, groan or grimace and withdraw the limb. With so-called *decorticate rigidity*, the arm slowly flexes and the leg extends. In *decerebrate rigidity*, which usually carries a worse prognosis than decorticate rigidity, the arms and legs extend, the back arches and the teeth clench. Both types of abnormal flexor and extensor response may be seen in structural, metabolic or toxic causes of coma. The pectoralis squeeze is valuable for comparing the two sides of the body to detect hemiparesis where one side fails to move, moves less than the other or postures abnormally (decorticate or decerebrate). Squeeze the medial side of the elbow, looking for abduction (good outcome) or adduction (bad outcome) of the shoulder; similarly, squeeze the medial side of the knee, where hip abduction with knee flexion is a

good sign, while adduction of the ipsilateral or often both hips, with extension of knee, is a bad sign. In some patients, it is hard to get any response, or nothing but a minor change in breathing, signifying deep coma, perhaps due to drug overdose. Ice water caloric stimulation (see the following) combined with the Doll's eye test may be used to demonstrate brainstem activity.

- The response of the pulse and blood pressure to painful stimuli may also be observed.

- **Caloric stimulation (oculovestibular reflex)**
  - This is usually done where brain death is suspected. The auditory canals are inspected (to exclude impacted wax or perforated drums), and the head elevated to 30 degrees above the horizontal. Then each external auditory canal is irrigated with iced water. In a normal conscious subject, this induces nystagmus with the fast component away from the ear. In coma, the fast component is lost and the eyes deviate towards the irrigated ear. In brain death, the reflex is lost. It may also be blocked by ototoxic drugs such as gentamycin, vestibular suppressant drugs such as phenytoin, and phenobarbitone and neuromuscular blockers.

The Glasgow coma scale

In the aftermath of a major neurological insult such as a head injury, it is important to monitor the level of coma, as this will determine whether further medical or surgical intervention is required. Its main use is for serial monitoring of a patient's neurological function, and does not replace a careful neurological assessment designed to evaluate the basis of a patient's coma and whether there is underlying focal pathology. The Glasgow Coma Scale scores the following items:

- Ability to open the eyes: 4, spontaneously; 3, to speech; 2, to pain; 1, none.

- Best motor response: 6, obeys commands; 5, localizes stimuli; 4, withdraws; 3, flexor posturing; 2, extensor posturing; 1, no movement.

- Best verbal response to stimulation: 5, orientated; 4, confused, inappropriate; 3, incomprehensible words; 2, sounds only; 1, none.

A comatose patient will have a score of 10 or less.

Some distinctive types of coma

- **Coma with myoclonic jerks/tremor.** This is seen in metabolic disorders such as diabetic coma, uraemia, hepatic failure and hypoxia. Other causes include hypoxic encephalopathy after prolonged cardiac arrest, CO_2 narcosis, high-dose intravenous penicillin or opiate encephalopathy and overdosage with selective serotonin reuptake inhibitors (SSRIs) causing serotoninergic toxicity.

- **Coma with roving eye movements**. These slow random movements of the eyes are commonly seen in persisting coma after cerebral anoxia or cardiac arrest and indicate an intact brainstem with diffuse cortical damage.

- **Coma with ocular bobbing**. Brisk downward bobbing movements of the eyes in this setting is associated with severe caudal pontine injury.

- **Coma with eyes deviated to one side:**
  - With a destructive lesion of one frontal lobe, the eyes will be deviated towards the side of the lesion. With an irritative acute lesion of one frontal lobe, as occurs transiently with cerebral haemorrhage (or in an adversive epileptic seizure), the eyes will be deviated away from the side of the lesion.
  - With a destructive lesion of the pons, the eyes will be deviated away from the side of the lesion.

- **Coma with eyes deviated downwards**. This is seen with thalamic haemorrhage or raised intracranial pressure from hydrocephalus (the 'sunset sign'), with the patient often appearing to be 'looking' at the tip of his nose. It is also associated with compression of the midbrain tectum and has been described in hepatic coma.

- **Coma with bilateral fixed dilated pupils**. This is a grave sign if persistent, usually associated with brain death. Other causes include overdosage with atropine-like drugs, severe barbiturate intoxication, hypothermia and transiently due to adrenalin injections during resuscitation.

- **Coma with one fixed dilated pupil**. In this setting, a fixed dilated pupil is due to a third nerve palsy resulting from coning or a ruptured posterior communicating aneurysm. If there is no ptosis or loss of eye movements, then it is more likely to be due to coning. Either way, this combination is an indication for urgent CT scanning.

- **Coma with pin-point pupils**. Consider opiate overdosage or pontine haemorrhage.

- **Coma with unilateral Horner's syndrome**. This is easily missed, as the only sign of it will be inequality of the pupils (best seen in dim light). Brush the back of your hand over the forehead on each side. If one side offers less resistance (because it is dry), and the pupil is smaller on that side, the patient has a Horner's syndrome. This is a good lateralizing but poor localizing sign. It is seen in hypothalamic and brainstem lesions. In a patient with a contralateral hemiplegia, dissection of the internal carotid is a consideration.

- **Coma with nystagmus**. Suspect epileptic activity – look for minor twitching of the corner of the mouth and perform an EEG. Look for spontaneous partial contraction and dilatation of the pupils (hippus).

● **Coma with hemiplegia.** Causes include contralateral cerebral haemorrhage, massive cerebral hemisphere infarction (as with internal carotid artery occlusion), bleeding or swelling of a tumour and subdural haematoma. An important treatable cause of this picture is hypoglycaemia (usually in a diabetic patient on oral agents or insulin).

● **Apparent coma with no response of the face or limbs to pain, nose tickle or corneal stimulation.** Ask the patient to look up and down. If they respond, they have the 'locked-in syndrome' usually due to an infarct or haemorrhage involving the pons. Vertical eye movements, a function of the midbrain, are spared.

● **Coma with a stiff neck.** Patients with generalized hypertonia may also have a stiff neck. A good working rule is that if the neck stiffness is due to meningism, it will only be on neck flexion that resistance is felt, not on neck rotation. Causes include subarachnoid haemorrhage, meningoencephalitis and coning from a supratentorial mass.

Box 14.1   Tips

● Always consider the possibility of reversible coma: hypoglycaemia (check the blood glucose, give intravenous glucose), non-convulsive epileptic status (perform an EEG) and opiate overdosage, which usually responds to naloxone.

● Small cerebral hemisphere lesions are not a cause of coma.

● Metabolic causes of coma usually do not affect the pupils or Doll's eye movements.

● Beware of performing a lumbar puncture in a comatose patient with a stiff neck – they may have raised intracranial pressure and be at risk of cerebral herniation. If bacterial meningitis is a serious consideration, start antibiotics while you conduct further tests, such as imaging.

15 Psychogenic (functional) neurological disorders

'Neurological' presentations of psychogenic disorders 122

It may seem surprising to be discussing psychogenic disorders in the context of the neurological examination. Surely, there will be no signs to find in a patient who does not have a neurological disease. Yet the difficulty of recognizing the signs of a psychogenic disorder should not be underestimated, and psychogenic disorders account for as many as 10–20 per cent of patients presenting to neurological clinics. The term 'functional neurological disorder' is now often used instead of psychogenic, but confusion can arise because the term functional is also sometimes used to denote 'organic' neurological disease where there is no obvious histological pathology (e.g. idiopathic dystonia), to denote neurosurgical procedures designed to alter function of the intact brain (functional neurosurgery), to denote special imaging (functional imaging) and to denote practitioners of alternative medicine (functional medicine). What matters is a clear, sympathetic and non-judgemental delivery of explanation of the diagnosis and management, whatever term is used.

Some general points about psychogenic disorders need to be made. This is an area where both the clinical skills and wisdom of the physician are most tested. Patients who have difficulty coping emotionally with a physical illness or who have unusual even bizarre presentations are too readily dismissed by the inexperienced physician as having psychogenic disorders. The opinion of a senior colleague here is invaluable. The label of 'psychogenic' must be applied with great caution, for thereafter, they may be treated as time wasters by unenlightened staff. It is not uncommon for patients with neurological disorders to develop psychogenic symptoms in addition to the organic disorder, particularly at times of stress. Very few patients with psychogenic disorders are true malingerers, and they deserve to be treated with kindness and compassion. These are the people in our society who are not coping with their lot.

Often the history, if the patient is willing to give it to you in full, is suggestive of a psychogenic disorder. Pointers include a history of sudden onset, many years of mysterious illnesses for which no definite cause can be found, multiple symptoms which cannot readily be explained by any disease process (somatiform disorder), periods of

DOI: 10.1201/9781003119166-15

severe disability alternating with periods of partial or complete spontaneous remissions or culminating in a sudden and dramatic 'cure' (as seen in 'faith healing'). It is the first psychogenic illness which poses the greatest diagnostic problem.

Until recently, neurologists were reluctant to make a firm diagnosis of psychogenicity for fear that eventually an organic basis for the symptoms would emerge. As a result, many patients were subjected to endless rounds of investigations, confirming their own worst fears about the nature of their illness, nor were they provided with the support and understanding which their condition required. Fortunately, the diagnosis of a psychogenic disorder is now widely accepted and respectable. When made by an experienced clinician it is rarely proven to be wrong.

'Neurological' presentations of psychogenic disorders

The key to recognising psychogenic illness is inconsistency and incongruence. Inconsistency refers to symptoms or signs that are not consistent with each other – e.g. the patient who cannot lift their legs from the bed during a formal neurological examination but can do so when asked to get out of bed. Incongruence refers to symptoms or signs that do not fit into known behaviour of organic disease – e.g. the patient with a diagnosis of Parkinson's disease who demonstrates significant weakness. For both inconsistency and incongruence, the challenge is to know the range of variation that can be observed in organic disease – e.g. the ability to walk backwards normally even if walking forwards is severely impaired in dystonia or the sudden evolution of dystonia-Parkinsonism that can occur with ATP1A3-related disease (rapid onset dystonia-Parkinsonism).

- **Gait.** Psychogenic gaits can come in many forms and include features such as knee-buckling, 'tight-rope' walking, 'collapses', convulsive shaking or extreme lurching and slowness. Many patients appear to be ataxic, but instead of compensating with a broad base, they walk with a narrow base and often even cross their feet while walking despite the appearance of extreme difficulties with balance ('astasia-abasia'). There may be emotive features such as exaggerated effort, sighing, groaning and gasping. Of course, all of these can happen in patients with a gait disturbance on an organic basis, but the difference is that in psychogenic gait there will be no relevant associated physical signs such as spasticity (increased tone and reflexes), clonus, rigidity, akinesia or intention tremor.

- **Tremor.** Psychogenic tremor is often dramatic, causing, for example, the arms to flap or the whole body to jig, and requiring so much exertion that the patient pants and sweats. As you watch, it may have a variable amplitude but also change its frequency, direction and distribution. If you engage the patient in conversation, it may momentarily cease altogether. Mentioning a particular limb may cause it to shake (*suggestibility*). Suggestibility may be also used to bring on a movement disorder that is paroxysmal and not present at the time of the evaluation. Thus, application of a tuning fork to the affected body part with the suggestion that 'vibration can cause an involuntary movement' often triggers the psychogenic movement. Likewise, a suggestion that 'vibration can stop an involuntary movement' often diminishes or completely suppresses the abnormal movement when a vibrating tuning fork is applied to the affected body part. Also, restraining the shaking limb may result in an emergence of shaking in contralateral limb or in another body part. Ask the patient to tap one hand in time with yours while you vary the frequency. If the tremor in the patient's other hand follows the rhythm that you are setting, this is called *entrainment* and is a feature of a psychogenic tremor. Asking the patient to perform the 'serial sevens' test or other mental task will often reduce the amplitude of psychogenic tremor or the tremor may cease completely. Parkinsonian or essential tremor, by contrast, increases during the 'serial sevens' test. The best *distraction* manoeuvre is to ask the patient to perform a complicated, sequential task with the opposite limb, such as repetitively touching the thumb with the second, fifth and then third finger of the same hand. These and other distraction manoeuvres will often cause psychogenic tremor to change its pattern or frequency, or cease. Unfortunately, some organic tremors may also be affected by distraction, so reliance should not be placed on this test alone.

- **Jerks**. Excessive startle is usually psychogenic. All of us jump in response to a loud noise or an unexpected pain, perhaps from a pin jab. These patients will 'jump out of their skin' in response to a tendon tap or a slight touch. Often they can be distracted from doing this by engaging them in conversation or by getting them to perform the 'serial sevens' test. Psychogenic startle has to be distinguished from the rare hyperekplexia and stimulus-sensitive or reflex myoclonus. The pattern of recruitment when recorded neurophysiologically often occurs in an orderly sequence, consistent with the normal anatomical distribution, in organic myoclonus whereas it is quite haphazard in psychogenic myoclonus. Also, when neurophysiological techniques are employed, latency from the stimulus (sudden loud sound or a visual threat) to the onset of muscle contraction is usually longer than 100 msec in psychogenic jerks whereas organic reflex myoclonus usually has a latency between 40 and 100 msec.

 See Video 107 Psychogenic tics
Psychogenic, distractable tics, precipitated by severe life stressors and triggered by suggestion and application of a tuning fork.

● **'Dystonia'**. Psychogenic dystonia, unlike most forms of dystonia, is usually manifested by fixed posture (i.e. cannot be overcome by passive movement). Although organic dystonia is rarely painful, patients with psychogenic dystonia often complain of painful spasms. When examining a patient with psychogenic dystonia, one often encounters resistance against passive movement. It may follow a minor injury and may be accompanied by discoloration of the skin and trophic changes, typically seen with reflex sympathetic dystrophy, now referred to as complex regional pain syndrome. Severe flexion of the spine (camptocormia) was first described in soldiers coming out of trenches during the First World War and found to be a feature of post-traumatic stress disorder. Although camptocormia may be psychogenic, there are many organic causes of camptocormia, such as Parkinson's disease and axial (trunk) dystonia.

● **Limb weakness**. Paralysis on a psychogenic basis often involves a single limb or the arm and leg on the same side. Features suggestive of this include excessive effort (grimacing, panting and gasping) when asked to move the affected limb(s), periods of days or weeks when power returns to normal, absence of objective signs such as changes in tone and reflexes or improvement with suggestion. A useful confirmatory sign in a patient with one 'paralysed' leg is the 'Hoover sign'. While lying on their back on the couch, ask them to raise the 'good' leg off the bed after you have placed your hand under the heel of the paralysed leg. You will feel a downward pressure from the otherwise completely paralysed leg.

● **Sensory loss**. This is very common, increasing in severity as the patient is subjected to repeated examinations in hospital. The key is that it does not conform to the anatomical boundaries of, say, a root or nerve. Rather, it will end at the top of the arm or top of the leg. With psychogenic 'hemisensory loss', the patient, unlike in an organic hemisensory loss, will not be able to feel the vibration of a tuning fork held on one side of the sternum but will be able to feel it on the other side (despite the fact that vibration is bilaterally conducted through the bone). Another test is to ask the patient to say 'yes' if they feel you touch them (with their eyes closed) or 'no' if they cannot. The timing of their response of 'no' after each touch tells you that they can feel it.

● **Speech/voice**
- Psychogenic speech disorders take a number of forms. One of the most common is *stutter* where whole words or phrases are repeated rather than the first sound, usually a consonant, of particular words, as occurs in organic stutter:
  - Psychogenic stutter: 'Drove drove drove down the road road road ...'
  - Organic stutter: 'D-D-D-Drove d-d-down the r-r-r-road ...'
- In organic stutter, the main feature is often 'blocking' where the patient cannot begin a sentence or gets stuck in the middle.

- Another type is *aphonia* where the patient can make no sound at all, nor mouth the words. Periods of normality are reassuring and help to confirm the diagnosis of psychogenicity. Reversion to child-like speech, acquisition of a foreign accent and the use of meaningless words ('neologism') are other examples of psychogenic speech.

● **Eyes/vision**

- A number of psychogenic disorders affecting the eyes and vision may be considered. Sudden complete *loss of all sight* including light perception is naturally very alarming – though often least so for the patient, who, paradoxically, may still be able to leave the house and go to work. Clues that this is psychogenic include the setting (often a young woman who is otherwise completely well), normal pupillary response to light (this, of course, can also occur with bilateral occipital infarction), inability to move the eyes voluntarily but preserved Doll's-eye movements, inability to point to where your voice is coming from (which can be readily done by hearing) or preserved menace response. Often sight returns spontaneously after a few days or weeks. 'Tunnel vision' is manifested by markedly narrowed field of peripheral vision when tested close and also when far (several yards) from the patient. *Convergence spasm* is often misdiagnosed as bilateral abducens palsies. Each eye appears to fail to abduct on either lateral gaze, producing markedly dysconjugate gaze with or without diplopia, accompanied by miosis (pupillary constriction). Although brainstem lesions can result in convergence spasm, this sign is often seen in the setting of psychogenic disorders. See Video 110.

See Video 108 Psychogenic nystagmus and opsoclonus

Intermittent tremor and intermittent multidirectional, conjugate gaze determined to be psychogenic nystagmus and opsoclonus.

See Video 109 Psychogenic convergence spasm

Psychogenic convergence spasm manifested by dysconjugate gaze and miosis and episodic left side 'involuntary' muscle contractions, triggered by a powerful suggestion and application of a vibrating tuning fork.

- *Pseudo-ptosis*, where the patient screws one eye up. Here, the eyebrow on the affected side is lowered, unlike in true ptosis where it is usually elevated (in an attempt to raise the eyelid). One exception is hemifacial spasm in which the ipsilateral eyebrow is often elevated due to frontalis contraction. This sign is also known as 'the other Babinski sign', described by Babinski to differentiate hemifacial spasm from blepharospasm in which the eyebrow is usually lowered.

Box 15.1 Tips

- Apparent indifference in the face of severe disability ('la belle indifference') is an unreliable marker of psychogenic disorders. It is, for example, commonly seen in the setting of multiple sclerosis.

- Psychogenic disorders are uncommon in children under the age of 6 years and should be diagnosed with caution when they occur for the first time in the elderly.

- The feature which often points to the possibility of a psychogenic disorder is the emotive, eye-catching quality of the presentation, sudden onset with spontaneous remissions, bizarre movement that is incongruous with organic movement disorder.

- The presence of undoubted psychogenic features does not exclude the possibility of an underlying physical illness.

- An absence of associated relevant objective physical signs, such as reflex changes, muscle wasting or cranial nerve lesions, is the starting point for making a diagnosis of a psychogenic disorder.

- Organic disorders where there are no associated signs accompanying the main feature are often misdiagnosed as psychogenic. These include dystonia, chorea and truncal ataxia (due to a midline cerebellar lesion where there may be no other cerebellar signs).

- The strongest evidence that a disorder has a psychogenic basis is a sudden onset, often triggered by recent stress, such as an argument, unresolved conflict or nonconsensual sexual encounter (e.g. rape or molestation). Lack of insight or denial of any stress prior to the onset of the symptoms is very frequent at the time of initial evaluation, and the psychodynamic factors may not be apparent until subsequent interviews.

- Sudden 'cure' – often triggered by suggestion, such as faith healing.

- The diagnosis of a psychogenic disorder must be based on 'positive' criteria, not merely the absence of organicity or negative investigation.

16 Telemedicine and the neurological examination

Introduction 127

The virtual neurological examination 128

Conclusions 130

Introduction

Telemedicine/telehealth examinations became widely used as a way of preventing the spread of infection during the COVID-19 pandemic which began in 2019. It was soon realized that there were other advantages to this type of assessment, in particular saving patients living in remote regions or with limited mobility the need to make their way to the clinic. But how did this type of assessment compare with the traditional assessment, especially in a discipline like neurology, which still places much emphasis on the clinical examination? Was it safe? Almost all published studies, including some randomized controlled trials, have confirmed the effectiveness of telehealth clinical assessments and outcomes when compared with face-to-face consultations.

Neurological disorders which can be assessed by taking a careful history, lend themselves particularly to telemedicine. These might include follow-up visits for epilepsy and other paroxysmal disorders such as headaches, but for most diseases, it is preferable for the assessment, especially the initial evaluation, to be done in the traditional way (face-to-face). It is probably unsuitable for disorders where diagnosis depends on eliciting neurological signs such as reflex changes, abnormal muscle tone and sensory loss. Where a formal neurological examination is required but it is not possible to conduct a face-to-face consultation, consider the option of engaging the assistance of a trained professional to attend the remote location with the patient to conduct the examination under your guidance.

The neurological history remains the cornerstone of the diagnostic process, and this is no different for a virtual neurological consultation. A good history allows a diagnostic formulation to be made before the neurological examination is conducted, which guides a hypothesis-driven examination. If anything, this is even more important if telemedicine is being used, as the examination is limited in its scope.

DOI: 10.1201/9781003119166-16

The virtual neurological examination

Positioning the patient and room requirements

In an ideal situation, a telemedicine consultation should be conducted in a well-lit room with the patient in a chair, facing the camera in a horizontal position with the microphone optimally activated. The patient should be close enough so that their face can be observed. The room should be large enough to assess stance and gait. It is preferable if someone else can be present to help the patient or to direct the camera.

Cognition and speech

Much of this will have been assessable during the history taking. During conversation with the patient, also observe for evidence of low volume voice or dysarthria. You may ask them to name body parts that you point to and make a brief mental status examination (orientation, memorizing three unrelated abjects after 5 minutes, subtract 7 from 100). For language, repetition can be easily tested. Simple verbal memory and word fluency can be tested. The patient can be asked to draw a cube and clockface to assess visuospatial function. In fact, much of the Minimental State Examination or Montreal Cognitive Assessment can be carried out remotely and correlates highly with face-to-face assessment if the patient is given pen and paper.

Cranial nerves

Gross visual acuity can be tested by asking the patient to count your fingers while covering each eye in turn. Major visual field loss and visual neglect can be determined by asking the patient when looking at your face on the screen, whether they can see both sides of the room clearly and also both sides of your face. Saccadic eye movements and range can be assessed by asking the patient to look from side to side, and up and down in the left lateral, right lateral and midline gaze positions. Look for nystagmus by asking the patient to maintain their eyes at the extremes of lateral and also midline vertical gaze. Downward eye movements can be difficult to assess because of the eyelids. Pursuit is difficult to assess, but the vestibulo-ocular reflex can be tested by asking the patient to turn their head from side to side at various speeds while looking at the camera. Facial symmetry and weakness are usually readily appreciated by asking the patient to close their eyes, smile and puff their cheeks out. Ask the patient then to open their mouth, looking for jaw deviation. Ask them to put their tongue out, looking for wasting, and to move it from side to side.

Upper limbs

Now ask the patient to move their chair back, so that you can see the upper half of their body. Ask them to lift both arms quickly to the horizontal, looking for lag of one arm which might indicate weakness or akinesia, or overshoot which might indicate limb ataxia. Ask them to close their eyes, looking for arm drift, and then with eyes closed, touch their nose with each index finger, which can give an indication of both intention tremor, but also proprioceptive loss. Ask them to perform fractionated finger movements (sequentially touching the tips of each of digits 2–5 to the tip of the thumb), which are disproportionately impaired in pyramidal lesions compared with flexing and extending all the fingers at the same time, even when power has returned to normal (see Chapter 2). Examine high-amplitude, rapid, repetitive movements with index finger touching the thumb, closing-opening of fists and supinating-pronating movements at the wrist. These repetitive movements are typically slow and have decrementing amplitude (with possible freezing) in patients with parkinsonism or are irregular in amplitude and rhythm in patients with ataxia (dysdiadochokinesis).

Lower limbs

Ask the patient to move their chair further back so that you can see the lower half of the body. While sitting, ask the patient to raise their knees by flexing their hips and observe for a "drift" while there are holding this position. Ask them to hold both legs straight out in front with knees extended, dorsiflex both feet and then alternately extend (dorsiflex) and flex (plantarflex) their feet at the ankle. While still in a sitting position, ask the patient to perform a heel-to-shin test. Also, ask the patient to repetitively tap the heels on the floor, looking for bradykinesia or dysdiadochokinesis. Now ask the patient to repetitively tap their toes loudly while keeping their heel grounded, looking for foot bradykinesia. These measures will detect severe and even moderate weakness. Then ask the patient to fold their arms and stand up, looking for proximal leg weakness or truncal ataxia.

Stance and gait

Now that the patient is standing, ask the patient to remove the chair and move back far enough so that you can see the whole body. Ask them to stand on their toes and heels, which is a further test of ankle strength. Ask the patient to walk towards and then away from the camera, preferably at least ten steps away from the camera, and then watch them turn and walk back at least six steps in tandem. There will be situations where a camera mounted to a computer or placed on a surface will not be able to capture stance and gait as described for logistical reasons. This is where the presence of a second person who can hold the camera can allow relocation to a more suitable space such as a hallway. If the patient is on their own and they are using a phone camera that cannot be placed in a static position that allows examination of stance and gait, if they have available a full-length mirror in a room with adequate space, ask the patient to position themselves an adequate distance from the mirror with the camera aimed at their reflection in the mirror. You can then examine their stance and gait while walking towards the mirror, although of course arm swing cannot be assessed with this manoeuvre.

Conclusions

Telemedicine and the virtual neurological examination have become part of standard clinical practice and should be embraced, while of course adhering to the requirements of local regulations. It offers major advantages to patients and carers. An awareness of its limitations and engagement of lay or professional assistants in the remote location during the telehealth consultation where needed will help overcome many issues. It cannot completely replicate the face-to-face consultation in many situations, especially the initial consultation or requirement for a full reassessment when an established patient has a new symptom. In this regard, it should be remembered that telemedicine is for the benefit of our patients, not the convenience of health professionals.

Picture credits

Figure 1.6   Adapted with permission from Figure 27 of *Aids to the Examination of the Peripheral Nervous System*, London, BaillièreTindall, 1986.

Figure 1.7   Adapted with permission from Figure 4.78a of Spillane JD and Spillane JA, *An Atlas of Clinical Neurology*, 3rd edn, Oxford, OUP, 1982.

Figure 1.8   Adapted with permission from Figure 76 of *Aids to the Examination of the Peripheral Nervous System*, London, BaillièreTindall, 1986.

Figure 1.9   Adapted with permission from Figure 36 of *Aids to the Examination of the Peripheral Nervous System*, London, BaillièreTindall, 1986.

Figure 1.11   Adapted with permission from Figure 87 of *Aids to the Examination of the Peripheral Nervous System*, London, BaillièreTindall, 1986.

Figure 2.1   Adapted with permission from Figure 15 of *Aids to the Examination of the Peripheral Nervous System*, London, BaillièreTindall, 1986.

Figure 2.3   Adapted with permission from Figure 72 of *Aids to the Examination of the Peripheral Nervous System*, London, BaillièreTindall, 1986.

Figure 3.1   Adapted with permission from Figure 11 of Jamieson EB, *Illustration of Regional Anatomy*, Section VI, Edinburgh, E& S Livingston.

Figure 3.2   Adapted with permission from Figure 1 of Jamieson EB, *Illustration of Regional Anatomy*, Section VI, Edinburgh, E& S Livingston.

Figure 4.1   Adapted with permission from Figure 46 of *Aids to the Examination of the Peripheral Nervous System*, London, Baillière Tindall, 1986.

Figure 5.1   Adapted with permission from Figure 4.34d of Spillane JD and Spillane JA, *An Atlas of Clinical Neurology*, 3rd edn, Oxford, OUP, 1982.

Figure 5.2   Adapted with permission from Figure 47 of*Aids to the Examination of the Peripheral Nervous System*, London, BaillièreTindall, 1986.

Figure 5.3   Adapted with permission from Figure 83 of *Aids to the Examination of the Peripheral Nervous System*, London, BaillièreTindall, 1986.

Figure 5.4   Adapted with permission from Figure 84 of *Aids to the Examination of the Peripheral Nervous System*, London, BaillièreTindall, 1986.

Figure 5.5   Adapted with permission from Figure 2.11 of Donaldson JO, *Neurology of Pregnancy*, 2nd edn, WB Saunders, 1989.

Figure 5.6   Adapted with permission from Figure 89 of *Aids to the Examination of the Peripheral Nervous System*, London, BaillièreTindall, 1986.

Figure 5.7   Adapted with permission from Figure 90 of *Aids to the Examination of the Peripheral Nervous System*, London, BaillièreTindall, 1986.

Figure 6.1   Adapted with permission from figures in Inman V, Human locomotion, *Canadian Medical Association Journal*, 1966;94: 1047–54.

Figure 6.2   Both adapted with permission from Figure 18.2 of Mumenthaler M, *Neurological Differential Diagnosis*, New York, Thieme-Stratton, 1985.

Index

Page numbers in *italics* refer figures and **bold** refer tables.

abducens nerve, palsy, *64*, 65
abductor pollicis brevis (APB), 2, *3*
abulia, 106, 113
acoustic neuroma, 49
Addenbrooke's Cognitive Examination, 110
    modified version, *111*
adductor digiti minimi (ADM), 2, *3*
Adie ('tonic') pupil, 71–72
age, of patient, 1
akathisia, 94
akinesia, 77
alcoholism, 72
Alzheimer's disease/syndrome, 110
ankle jerk, absence of, 31
apathy, 106
aphasia, 97–98, 100–104
    current definitions, **103**
aphonia, 125
apraxia
    dressing, 18
    of eyelid opening, 90
    miming in, 112
    in Parkinson's disease, 112
Argyll Robertson (A-R) pupil, 72
arms
    dermatomes, *7*
    'flail' arm, 7
    most useful muscles to test, xxvi
    proximal weakness, 14–21
    screening tests, xxix; *see also* wrist drop
Arnold-Chiari malformation, 70
arthritis, 1, 25; *see also* osteoarthritis
asterixis, 86
ataxia, 33–43; *see also* Friedreich's ataxia
ataxic nystagmus, 70
athetosis, 88, 90
attention, 106

bat's wing tremor, 81
behaviour, and dementia, 106–108
Bell's palsy, 44, 47–50
    and hearing, 51
    and hypertension, 52
'Benediction sign', 3, *4*, 5
Benedict's syndrome, 53

bilateral ptosis, 56–57
birth trauma, 2
blepharospasm, 90
blood pressure, swings, 106
brachioradialis, *13*, 20
bradykinesia, 112
brainstem
    lesions, 50
    myoclonus, 87
breathing patterns, altered, 106
Brown-Séquard syndrome, 31
bruising, 105–106
bruxism, 95
buttocks, dermatomes, *30*

caloric stimulation, and coma assessment, 118
camptocormia, 124
    dystonic, 42
central visual field, testing, 60, *60*
cerebellar dysfunction, signs of, 74–82
cerebellar nystagmus, 69
cerebral haemorrhage, 119
cervical dystonia, gait, 41
cervical spondylosis, 9
C5/6, muscles supplied by, *17*
Charcot-Marie-Tooth disease, 27, 35
chorea, 82, 84, 96
    in Huntington's disease, 91
clawing, of ring and little fingers, 2
cognitive impairment, 105
cognitive testing, formal, 109–110
coma, 115
    assessment, 115–120
    reversible, 120
common peroneal nerve
    lesion, 27, *29*, 35
    muscles supplied by, *29*
complete ptosis, 57
CO_2 narcosis, 118
conjugate gaze, palsy, 66
consciousness, level of, 106
convergence-retraction nystagmus, 71
convergence spasm, 73
    psychogenic, 125
coordination, xxvii

copropraxia, 85
corneal reflex, and coma assessment, 117
cortical myoclonus, 87
cough, 99
cough reflex, and coma assessment, 117
cover test, 62
Creutzfeldt-Jakob disease, 113
cylindroma, 45

declarative memory, 114
delirium, vs dementia, 105–106
dementia, 105
    vs delirium, 105–106
    frontal lobe type, 110, 112–113
    frontotemporal, 107
    with Lewy bodies, 112
    in parkinsonism, 110, 112
    vascular, 113
dermatomyositis, 15
diabetes mellitus, 7
    adult-onset, 25
diagnosis formulation, xxx
diplopia, confirmation of, 62
disinhibition, 106
distraction manoeuvres, 123
doll's eye movements, 62
    and coma assessment, 116–117
dopa-induced involuntary movements,
    92–93
dopamine-receptor blocking drugs *see*
    neuroleptics
dorsiflexion, weakness, 28, 30
drowsiness, 8, 106
dysarthria, 97–100
    progressive, 40
dyskinesia
    dopa-induced, 42, 91, 93
    tardive, 94–95
dysmetria, 79
dysrhythmia, 79
dysthyroid eye disease, 72
dystonia, 87–88, 96
    beginning/end-of-dose, 93
    blepharospasm/cranial, 92
    craniocervical, 89, 95
    generalized, 88, 92
    oromandibular, 95
    progressive generalized, 42
    psychogenic, 124
    tardive, 95–96
    task-specific, 89

tremor syndromes, 79–80; *see also* cervical
    dystonia; torsion dystonia
dystonia-Parkinsonism, 122
dystrophia myotonica *see* myotonic dystrophy

Eaton-Lambert syndrome, 25
encephalopathy
    hypoxic, 118
    metabolic, 104
    opiate, 119
    Wernicke's, 70
entrainment, 123
environmental dependence, 106
epileptic seizure, adversive, 119
epileptic status, non-convulsive, 120
episodic memory, 114
essential tremor, 76, 82
eversion, weakness, 28, 30
executive dysfunction, 106
eyelid drooping *see* ptosis
eye movement
    abnormalities, 58–73
    testing, 61–62
eye muscles, weakness, 64–66

face, 15
    bilateral weakness, 51
    screening tests, xxix
    swelling, 51
    weakness, 44–52
facial nerve
    course and relations, 45
    lesion, *46*
fasciculations, 2, 15, 27
    generalized, 9
femoral nerve, muscles supplied by, *24*
fingers, abduction, *3*
first dorsal interosseous (1st DI), 2, *3*
'flail' arm, 7
Fleischer, Richard, 80
fluent aphasia, 97, 101–104
foot drop, 26–32
Friedreich's ataxia, 27
frontal lobe type dementia, 110, 112–113
frontal meningioma, 113
fundi, and coma assessment, 116
fundoscopy, 59

gag reflex, and coma assessment, 117
gait, 26, 78
    antalgic, 42–43

ataxic, 40
broad-based, *34*
cerebellar, 40
'dancing', 41
disturbance, 33–43
hemiparetic, 27, 37
high-stepping, 34–35
normal, *34*
parkinsonian, 38
psychogenic, 122
scissoring, 37
shuffling, 43
spastic, 35, 38
waddling, 36–37
wide-based unsteady, 79
gaze-evoked nystagmus, 69
geniculate herpes, 45
Gerstmann's syndrome, 104
Glasgow coma scale, 118
glioma, 50
Gowers' sign, 23
grasping, 113
    forced, 106, 108
grasp reflex, 107
grooming, 105
groping, 107, 113
    forced, 106
Guillain-Barré syndrome, 22, 47
    Miller Fisher variant, 51

hand length, 2; *see also* wasted hand
head drop, 20
hearing, 51
hemianopia, bitemporal, 63
hemiatrophy, 2
hemiballismus, 84
hemifacial spasm, 44
    post-Bell's, 49
hemiparesis, 31, 84
    homonymous, 63
hemiplegia, and coma assessment, 120
hemisensory loss, psychogenic, 124
hepatic failure, 118
higher cortical function, testing, 105–114
hips
    congenital dislocation, 37
    flexion, weakness, 30
Holmes-Adie syndrome, 72
Holmes tremor, 80
horizontal nystagmus, 69, 71
Horner's syndrome, 1–2, *54*, 55, 57, 71

and coma assessment, 119
Huntington's disease
    and chorea, 91
    gait, 41
    and voluntary gaze, 61
hydrocephalus, 32, 119
    normal pressure, 113
hyperacusis, 51
hypoglycaemia, 120
hypomimia, 48
hypothyroidism, 113
hypoxia, 118

imitation behaviour, 108
impulsiveness, 106
incongruence, 122
inconsistency, 122
infection, 106
inspection, xxvi
intention tremor, 76–77, 79
internuclear ophthalmoplegia (INO), 2, *64*,
    66, 70
inversion, weakness, 28

jaw jerk, and coma assessment, 117
jerks, psychogenic, 123
joints, 15
    shoulder, *16*

Kayser, Bernard, 80
Kearns-Sayre syndrome, 54, 56
knee flexion, weakness, 30

language, 106
    disturbance, 97–104
    main areas, *101*
laryngeal myoclonus, 87
lateral gaze, pathway, *67*
legs
    dermatomes of lower leg, *30*
    most useful muscles to test, xxvii
    proximal weakness, 22–25
    screening tests, xxix
    spasticity, 32
    spastic weakness of, 8
leprosy, 50
levodopa, 92–93
L4/5, lumbosacral cord arising from, *29*
limb reflexes, and coma assessment, 117
limb weakness, psychogenic, 124
'liver flap', 86

locked-in syndrome, 120
'loss of check', 79
Luria's test, 112

Machado-Joseph disease, 40
marche à petits pas, 39
Marcus Gunn response, 61
median nerve
   lesion, 2
   muscles supplied by, *4*
   sensory distribution, *5*
Melkersson-Rosenthal syndrome, 51
memory, 114
Meniere's disease, 69
metabolic disturbance, 106
Miller Fisher syndrome, 57
mimicry, forced *see* imitation behaviour
Mini-Mental State Examination (MMSE),
      110, 113
   remote, 128
mini-myoclonus, 87, 91
Montreal Cognitive Assessment (MoCA), 110,
      113
   remote, 128
motor neurone disease (MND), 2, 8, 22, 35, 48
   diagnosis, 9
   split hand in, *2*
mouth grasp, 107
multiple sclerosis, 71
   and facial palsy, 51
multiple system atrophy (MSA),
      progressive, 81
muscle power, xxvi
muscle weakness, generalized, 8
muscular dystrophy, 37
myasthenia gravis, 48, 55–56, 72
   ocular, 57
myoclonus, 82, 86–87, 96
myoclonus-dystonia syndrome, 89
myopathy, 37, 48
   ocular, 56
myorhythmia, 81
myotonic dystrophy, 8–9, 48, 56

neck, stiffness, 120
negative myoclonus, 86
neologism, 101
neuroleptics, 93–94
neuropathy, peripheral, 8, 28
non-fluent aphasia, 100–101, 103
nose tickle, and coma assessment, 117

nystagmus, 68–72
   and coma assessment, 119
   psychogenic, 125

obturator nerve, muscles supplied by, *24*
oculocephalic reflex *see* doll's eye movements
oculomotor nerve, palsy, *54*, *55*, 65
oculovestibular reflex *see* caloric stimulation
ophthalmoplegia, bilateral, 51
optic disc, swelling, 72
optic nerve, disease, 72
optic neuritis, 72
osteoarthritis, of hips, 37
'other Babinski sign', 126
overdose
   drug or alcohol, 106
   opiate, 120
overshoot *see* dysmetria

painful stimuli responses, and coma
      assessment, 117–118
palatal myoclonus, 87
Pancoast tumour, 7
paralysis, psychogenic, 124
paraparesis, 30
paraphasia, 101
parasagittal tumours, 31
Parinaud's syndrome, 67–68, 71
parkinsonism
   and dementia, 110, 112
   drug-induced, 96
   and tremor, 75
Parkinson's disease, 81
   apraxia, 112
   arthritis, 1
   falls, 78
   gait, 38, 43
   lack of facial expression, 48
   speech, 78
   tremor, 75–78, 82
pattern recognition, 83
pendular nystagmus, 71
penicillin, high-dose intravenous, 118–119
percussion myotonia, 8
peripheral nystagmus, 69
peripheral visual field, testing, 59–60, *59*
pes cavus, 27, *28*, 31
physiological tremor, 76
plantar responses, and coma assessment, 117
polio, 2
pons, transverse section, *45*

pontine metastasis, 66
post-hypoxic myoclonus, 86
postural tremor, 76, 78–79
power, coordination and reflexes, 3–8
primary gaze position, testing, 61
primary writing tremor, 74
procedural memory, 114
progressive supranuclear palsy (PSP), 61–62, 68, 112
pseudobulbar palsy, 48
pseudo-dementia, 113
pseudoptosis, 126
psychogenic disorders, 121–126
ptosis, 50–51, 53–57
'pull test', 39, 78
pupils, 1
    abnormalities, 71–72
    and coma assessment, 116, 119
    testing responses, 61
pursuit gaze, testing, 62

quadrantanopia, upper/lower homonymous, 64

radial nerve
    lesion, 10, 12
    muscles supplied by, 11
Ramsay Hunt syndrome, 45
receptive aphasia, 97
reflexes, xxvii–xxviii
reflex myoclonus, 86
resting tremor, 75, 77
Rinné test, 69
Romberg's sign, 35–36, 43
rotator cuff injuries, 20, 21

saccadic gaze, testing, 61–62
sarcoidosis, 45, 47
scars, on arms, 2
sciatic nerve, lesion, 30
screening tests, xxix
selective serotonin reuptake inhibitors (SSRIs), overdose, 119
semantic memory, 114
senile ptosis, 56–57
sensory loss, psychogenic, 124
sensory testing, xxviii
serotoninergic toxicity, 119
serratus anterior
    mode of action on scapula, 15
    weakness, 19

skin, 15
    cancer, 48–49
slow tremor see myorhythmia
somatosensory evoked potentials (SSEPs), 87
speech
    disturbance, 97–104
    in Parkinson's disease, 78
    psychogenic disorders, 124–125
spina bifida, 27
spinal myoclonus, 87
spine, lower, 27
startle, psychogenic, 123
Steele Richardson syndrome, 62, 68
stereotypies, 90, 95
stroke, 2, 37, 44, 47
    facial numbness, 49
suggestibility, 123
supinator, inverted, 17
sweating, 106
synkinesis, 45–46, 49
syringobulbia, 50

tachycardia, 106
tardive syndromes, 93–96
taste, 50
technique, xxv–xxx
telehealth examinations, 127
telemedicine, 127–130
third nerve, palsy, 53, 57, 71
thumb, abduction, 3
tics, 82, 85, 96
    psychogenic, 123
tone, xxvi, 77
    and coma assessment, 117
torsion dystonia, gait, 41
torticollis, 88, 92
Tourette's syndrome, 85, 91
trapezius
    mode of action on scapula, 15
    weakness, 19
tremor, 74–82
    drug-induced, 96
    psychogenic, 122–123
Trendelenburg's test, 36, 36, 43
trigeminal nerve, lesions, 50
trochlear nerve, palsy, 64, 66
tunnel vision, 125

ulnar nerve
    lesions, 2, 6
    muscles supplied by, 6

sensory distribution, 5
trauma, 2
unilateral ptosis, 55–56
uraemia, 118
utilization behaviour, 108, 113

vascular dementia, 113
vertical nystagmus, 70
vestibular nystagmus, 68–69
virtual neurological examination, 128–130
vision
abnormalities, 58–73
psychogenic disorders, 125
visual acuity
impairment in one eye, 63
testing, 58–59
visual field

losses and associated lesions, 63
testing, 59–60
Vitamin B$_{12}$ deficiency, 113

wasted hand, 1–9
wasting, 15, 27
of both hands, 8
distal, 8
distribution, 2
of one hand, 7–8
Weber test, 69
Wernicke's aphasia, 97, 102
Wilson's disease, 80–81
wing-beating tremor, 80
working memory, 114
wrist drop, 10–13
radial deviation, 12

Printed in the United States
by Baker & Taylor Publisher Services